INSTRUMENTATION
FOR
EYECARE
PARAPROFESSIONALS

INSTRUMENTATION FOR EYECARE PARAPROFESSIONALS

Michelle Pett Herrin, CO, COMT

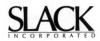 The Basic Bookshelf for Eyecare Professionals

Series Editors Janice K. Ledford, COMT • Ken Daniels, OD • Robert Campbell, MD

SLACK INCORPORATED   6900 Grove Road, Thorofare, NJ 08086

Publisher: John H. Bond
Editorial Director: Amy E. Drummond
Assistant Editor: Elisabeth DeBoer

Herrin, Michelle Pett.
    Instrumentation for eyecare paraprofessionals/Michelle Pett Herrin.
      p. cm. -- (The basic bookshelf for eyecare professionals)
    Includes bibliographical references and index.
    ISBN 1-55642-399-3 (alk. paper)
    1. Ophthalmology--Equipment and supplies. 2. Optometry--Equipment and supplies.
3. Opticianry--Equipment and supplies. 4. Ophthalmic assistants. I. Title. II. Series.
    [DNLM: 1. Ophthalmology--instrumentation. 2. Diagnostic Equipment. 3. Ophthalmic Assistants. WW 26H5671 1998]
    RE73.H45 1998
    617.7'0028--dc21
    DNLM/DLC
    for Library of Congress   98-38796
                                                                                                CIP

Published by: SLACK Incorporated
                     6900 Grove Road
                     Thorofare, NJ 08086-9447 USA
                     Telephone: 609-848-1000
                     Fax: 609-853-5991
                     World Wide Web: http://www.slackinc.com

Contact SLACK Incorporated for more information about other books in this field or about the availability of our books from distributors outside the United States.

Authorization to photocopy items for internal or personal use, or the internal or personal use of specific clients, is granted by SLACK Incorporated, provided that the appropriate fee is paid directly to Copyright Clearance Center, 222 Rosewood Drive, Danvers, MA 01923 USA, 978-750-8400. Prior to photocopying items for educational classroom use, please contact the CCC at the address above. Please reference Account Number 9106324 for SLACK Incorporated's Professional Book Division.

For further information on CCC, check CCC Online at the following address: http://www.copyright.com.

Last digit is print number: 10 9 8 7 6 5 4 3 2 1

Dedication

To the cutest piano and soccer player who is getting ready for junior high school.
Michael, you are the light of my life.

Contents

    General Considerations

    General Considerations in the Exam Room

    OSHA Standards

    HIV in the Eyecare Practice

    Projectors

    Projector Slides

    Screens

    Front Surface Mirrors

    Distance and Near Vision Charts

    Brightness Acuity Tester (BAT)

    Vision Screener

    HRR Color Blindness Plates and Ishihara Color Deficiency Test Books

    Farnsworth Dichotomous 15 and 100 Hue

    Optokinetic Drum and Tape

    Photoscreening Devices

    Phoropter

    Autorefractor

    Streak or Spot Retinoscope

    Lensmeter

    Automatic Lensmeter

    Trial Frame

    Trial Lenses

    Cross Cylinder

    Distometer

    Loose Prisms

    Prism Bar

    Rotary or Risley Prism

    Stereopsis Tests

    Maddox Rod

    Worth 4 Dot

    Bagolini Lenses

Acknowledgments

There are several people I would like to thank, because without their help this book could not have been written.

J. Brad Santora	Marco Technologies Inc, Jacksonville, Florida
Karen Amyot	Volk Optical, Inc, Mentor, Ohio
Ted Rzemien	Hilco® Inc, Plainville, Massachusetts
Marcus Dangeli	Haag-Streit, Koeniz, Switzerland
Melody Bertolucci and Gina Crabb	Zeiss Humphrey Systems, Dublin, California
Eric and Pam Larsen	Larsen Equipment Design Inc, Seattle, Washington
David Biggens and Linda Hausen	Leica/Reichert, Buffalo, New York
Tracy Heiss	AIT Industries, Elmhurst, Illinois
Rae Ann Bird	Mentor® 0&0 Inc, Santa Barbara, California
Robert Brennen	Medical Technologies & Innovations Inc, Lancaster, Pennsylvania
Donna Martin	Titmus Optical Inc, Petersburg, Virginia

I need to give special thanks to my employer, Michaelis Jackson, MD (the World's Greatest Eye Doctor), and two super techs, Donna and Cheryl, for allowing me to try all of this out in our office. Also thanks to La Rue Sumner and Carolyn Stull for their help.

I wish to thank Rhonda Curtis, CRA, COT for writing the maintenance on the fundus camera, and for her last minute photographs. I took my last fundus photo 20 years ago! Rhonda is the Director of Ophthalmic Photography at Washington University School of Medicine in St. Louis and the JCAHPO representative for the Ophthalmic Photography Society (OPS). She lives in St. Louis with her two daughters, Vanessa and Valenda, and her two dogs, Pepper and Katie.

I could not have done this without two very special people, (the most obvious) Mom and Dad. And last but not least, to Jan Ledford, my editor—where would I be without your red pen? I could not have completed this project without all of the above mentioned family and friends.

About the Author

Michelle Pett Herrin, CO, COMT, began her career in ophthalmic medical technology in Michigan in 1973 when she learned to grind spectacle lenses. She later attended the University of Florida's Ophthalmic Technician/Orthoptic Program where she earned her credentials. She subsequently started the first Bachelor of Science Program for Ophthalmic Technology at Wayne State University in Detroit. As a member of the Association of Technical Personnel in Ophthalmology (ATPO) since 1977, she currently serves as a commissioner to the Joint Commission on Allied Health Personnel in Ophthalmology (JCAHPO). She has taught continuing education classes for JCAHPO, and has moderated for ATPO's Scientific Session. She is currently the secretary of the JCAHPO Research and Education Foundation, and has been a director of the Foundation since 1991.

Instrumentation for Eyecare Paraprofessionals is Michelle's second book. Her previous book, *Ophthalmic Examination and Basic Skills*, has been used by some training programs as an introduction to ophthalmic assisting. In 1982 Michelle moved to Harrisburg, Illinois (in the middle of coal mines and corn fields) with her husband Roger, son Michael, and puppy dog Buddy. Dr. Michaelis Jackson, her sponsoring ophthalmologist, opened a satellite office in Michelle's hometown and she has the luxury of walking to work. Michelle is a trustee on the local library board, and is a director on the board of a clinic that provides free medical care for all of southern Illinois. Michelle claims she is a "soccer mom" who actually lives in her car, since soccer and piano practice are a one hour drive away.

Foreword

There are three keys to a successful eyecare practice:
1) technology and equipment
2) support staff and personnel
3) integration of the supporting staff's professional education and actual clinical experience.

Of these three cornerstones, training and education of support staff/personnel is the most critical foundation to any practice. Without the knowledge and understanding of the various instruments utilized in the eyecare field, support staff will not be able to adequately assist an ophthalmologist or optometrist in a clinical setting.

So often new personnel are met with an enormous amount of material to assimilate and learn, including new vocabulary, new techniques, and new equipment. Most of the inexperienced are overwhelmed and consumed with rote memorization of terms and techniques that hamper their ability to truly master the procedures and protocols necessary to better assist the practitioner.

This book contains valuable information on how to identify and maintain the essential equipment needed to provide quality patient care. Every support staff member, no matter what his or her level of experience, will find this manual to be a useful guide through the ever-evolving dynamics of eyecare equipment and its maintenance.

In addition, instrument maintenance is included in all exams for ophthalmic and optometric certification exams. This book will aid certification candidates in preparing for their exams.

This book will help your office work better and smarter because quality eyecare cannot be performed if equipment malfunctions.

Michaelis Jackson, MD
Director, Department of Ophthalmology, Carbondale Clinic, Carbondale, Illinois
Chief, Surgical Ophthalmology, Veterans Administrations Hospital, Marion, Illinois
Associate Clinical Professor, Southern Illinois University School of Medicine, Carbondale, Illinois

Preface

When I first started this book, I was told that if an instrument was not working, the cleaning crew had probably unplugged it overnight! This statement is somewhat true considering that equipment manufactured today has become very solid and efficient. Proper use along with regular maintenance keeps instruments in top working condition. Regular maintenance is essential for outstanding performance and if followed properly, problems will rarely occur.

There are many manufacturers of eyecare equipment. The instruments that are covered in this book are the ones I chose because they are currently in our office. Always refer to maintenance manuals when unsure of proper procedures.

Improvements and changes in equipment are constantly occurring. These improvements make the job we do as eyecare paraprofessionals easy and efficient.

Editor's Note: The purpose of this book is to describe the use and maintenance of instruments used in eyecare. For specific how-to's of instrument use, please consult appropriate Basic Bookshelf Series titles such as Basic Procedures, A Systematic Approach to Strabismus, The Slit Lamp Primer, etc.

The Study Icons

The *Basic Bookshelf for Eyecare Professionals* is quality educational material designed for professionals in all branches of eyecare. Because so many of you want to expand your careers, we have made a special effort to include information needed for certification exams. When these study icons appear in the margin of a *Series* book, it is your cue that the material next to the icon (which may be a paragraph or an entire section) is listed as a criteria item for a certification examination. Please use this key to identify the appropriate icon:

OptA	optometric assistant
OptT	optometric technician
OphA	ophthalmic assistant
OphT	ophthalmic technician
OphMT	ophthalmic medical technologist
LV	low vision subspecialty
Srg	ophthalmic surgical assisting subspecialty
CL	contact lens registry
Optn	opticianry
RA	retinal angiographer

Note: Most Basic Bookshelf Series titles contain a patient education sidebar (boxed material) entitled "What the Patient Needs to Know." Because of the technical nature of the material in Instrumentation for Eyecare Paraprofessionals, the sidebar will not appear.

Chapter 1

General Preventative Maintenance

KEY POINTS

- Maintain equipment records and manuals.

- Keep equipment covered or properly stored at night.

- Turn illuminated equipment off when not in use.

- Follow accepted cleaning and maintenance procedures.

- Use a rechargeable instrument all day long—do not recharge in-between use.

General Considerations

Properly functioning equipment is of utmost importance in the eyecare practice. Patient care runs more smoothly when instruments and equipment are in top working condition and can obtain accurate data. Care, maintenance, calibration, and simple repairs of equipment (as well as knowledgeable personnel who can perform these tasks) are necessary in a well-run practice. Knowledge and understanding of all equipment can prevent loss of patient care time and prevents a patient from having to return to the office. Accurate calibration provides reliable data and helps prevent errors in data collection. In addition, instrument maintenance and repair is needed to pass certification and registration exams in both ancillary ophthalmic and optometric professions.

Maintenance Manuals

A maintenance manual should be kept to record an instrument's name, model number, serial number, age, and current phone numbers of the company or its service representative. Keep a list of all replacement parts and their numbers. In addition, keep phone numbers of suppliers of consumables (bulbs, fuses, chin papers, etc) and the product number, as well as standard alternatives. Often these alternatives can be less costly to the practice. An adequate supply of consumable products should be kept on hand to maintain continuous use. Keep all manuals and supplies in a convenient and central location.

When a new piece of equipment comes in, the information mentioned above should be recorded. Learn how to care for and maintain the new instrument from the manufacturer's representative if possible. Read the manual provided with the instrument, especially the maintenance portion. If possible, more than one person in the practice needs to understand how to care for the new instrument.

Standard Tools

Minor repairs often need a set of screwdrivers (including small jewelers and Phillips head), Allen wrenches, and a small nut driver set. Adjustable pliers (including needlenose), electricity testers, and electrical tape are also valuable basic tools that should be kept on hand. Specialized tools often accompany a new piece of equipment. Keep these tools in a safe and central location or with the instrument itself.

General Cleaning and Disinfection

The most important step in cleaning equipment is to keep it covered at night with an appropriate cover or properly store it in its container. Most external surfaces of instruments are painted metal, plastic, or vinyl. These can be dusted with a soft cloth. The cloth can be used dry or with a spray. Never directly spray an instrument with any type of cleaner; always spray it on the cleaning cloth. Before attempting to dust an instrument, check the manufacturer's specifications so that surfaces are not damaged by a cleaner that is too harsh. Canned air or cotton-tipped swabs can be used to clean small areas or crevices that cannot be reached by dusting (Figure 1-1). Care should be taken when using canned air, because tilting some cans may cause the gas to be dispensed as a cold moist liquid which could possibly alter the appearance of some plastics and other materials. A black plastic surface takes on a milky white appearance when canned air is not used properly.

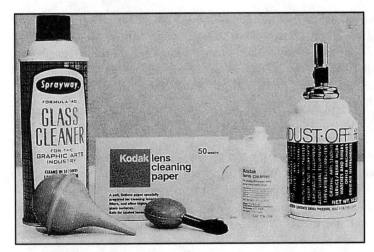

Figure 1-1. Compressed air, a camel hair brush, optical lens cleaners, and lens tissues are essential in cleaning sensitive eyecare equipment. (Reprinted from Blair B, Appleton B, Garber N, Crowe M, and Alven M. *Opticianry, Ocularistry and Ophthalmic Technology.* Thorofare, NJ: SLACK Incorporated; 1990.)

Extreme but very simple care is necessary when cleaning lenses or front surfaced mirrors. Never use tissue, paper towels, or any cloth that will scratch the surface. Some lenses are glass, while others are plastic. Lenses may be "bloomed" or specially coated to reduce reflections. Cleaning with improper cloths or solvents can result in immediate damage to the lens surface. Always check the lens type and manufacturer's cleaning instructions before attempting to clean any lens surface.

Some important things to keep in the office for lens cleaning are good photographic lens wipes, a soft linen cloth that is lint free, canned air, and cleaning solutions. Some cleaning solutions for glass lenses are a mixture of four parts ether to one part isopropyl alcohol, or one part ammonia to one part isopropyl alcohol. A glass cleaner can be used on some glass lenses. A bloomed lens should never be wiped in a dry state, but may be cleaned with either 100% ethyl or methyl alcohol on a clean lens wipe. Contact lens cleaning solutions are great for cleaning some plastic lenses. Whatever cleaning method or solution that is used should be used very sparingly and very carefully. Too much solution can ruin seals and possibly the lens itself.

A front surfaced mirror has a silver coating on the front surface of the glass so that light is bounced directly off of the silver coating. A pencil tip touched lightly to a front surface mirror will show the pencil lead and its reflection touching each other. A pencil tip touched to the surface of a back surface mirror will show a space between the tip and its reflection. This space is the thickness of the glass. The silver coating on a front surface mirror can easily be damaged if not cared for properly. Canned air or a camel hair brush will remove light debris and dust. Special solutions can be used, but these should be used infrequently because the mirror's surface will rub off slightly with each cleaning.

Any instrument that has contact with more than one patient must be properly cleaned, disinfected, or sterilized. Isopropyl alcohol wipes are very convenient on most surfaces. Solutions of one part household bleach to ten parts water or 3% hydrogen peroxide are good disinfectants. Chemicals and cleaning solutions must always be thoroughly rinsed from any surface that may contact a patient's eye before the instrument is used.

General Considerations of Bulbs

Most of the illuminated equipment used in eyecare does not contain a fan for air cooling. Consequently there is heat buildup which ultimately shortens a bulb's life. Therefore, it is important to turn off all illuminated equipment immediately after use. A backup supply of bulbs should be maintained so that a blown bulb can be replaced immediately. A bulb's jacket should never be touched. (This is true of all light bulbs, even the ones in your home.) The oil from your fingers will not only shorten the bulb's life, but the fingerprint can be etched into the glass jacket and cause a shadow in the illumination field. A glass jacket can be wiped with lens tissue or a soft cloth if you suspect that the bulb may have fingerprints on it. A decrease or change in the size or shape of an illumination field can be caused by an overheated bulb or from a bulb that was left on for a long period of time.

When changing a bulb, turn off and unplug the instrument. Do not attempt to remove a hot bulb—wait until it is cool before you remove it. A bulb may screw in, push straight in, or it may be pushed in and then turned. Some bulbs may not blow out, but do not give off enough illumination to achieve proper calibration. Some bulbs can be rotated 180 degrees and offer two sides of illumination. These types of bulbs should be rotated on a regular basis, extending the life of the bulb.

General Considerations of Power Supplies

Power sources include wall sockets, transformers, and rechargeable and standard batteries. In eyecare practice a great majority of instruments are hand-held or portable. Standard batteries are used in some, for example the Worth 4 Dot, while rechargeable batteries are used in others, such as most retinoscopes or ophthalmoscopes. Standard batteries should be removed from a piece of equipment if it will not be in use for some time. Removing these batteries will help prevent corrosion. Keep extra batteries stored in the refrigerator or freezer. This can help extend the life of the battery.

An instrument with a rechargeable battery should be used all day long without placing it into the charger instead of recharging between each use. It should be left in the recharger overnight for the next day's use. Rechargeable batteries have memories, and operating time diminishes dependent upon time of use and time spent in the charger. Operating time will decrease if the rechargeable instrument is constantly placed in the charger between uses. If this happens, the life of the battery is shortened and the instrument will not work all day without recharging between use.

Some instruments use transformers. Cords connect the instrument to its power source. Always make sure that these cords are not defective or loose, and that the contacts are not corroded. Corroded contacts can be cleaned. Depending upon the amount of corrosion involved, a pencil eraser or file can be used to clean contacts. Don't always assume that wall sockets are working, because they too, can be defective. If an instrument will not turn on, make sure it is plugged in before attempting any heroic repairs. Cleaning crews sometimes unplug an instrument. Surge protectors are valuable to help protect computerized equipment. This small inexpensive device can save sensitive equipment from voltage fluctuations.

A fuse is like a light bulb that does not produce light. It has a filament in a glass jacket that helps regulate electrical currents in the instrument. If the electrical current is overloaded the fuse will blow. This protects the instrument. A fuse can be replaced easily by turning the instrument off and inserting a new fuse. Read manufacturer's guidelines for proper amperage. An amp that is too low will not carry the electrical load, whereas an amp that is too high can damage the instrument.

General Considerations in the Exam Room

A clean, well-stocked exam room is important in maintaining eye equipment and instruments. The room should be ready for use at all times. The location of the office (for example if it is located near a factory), smoking, and open windows can contribute to increased air pollution. Clean air is important in the eyecare exam room. Air purifiers can be beneficial to remove airborne dust, lint, and small pollutants (bacteria, mold, and fungi). Some units can even help to reduce static electricity.

The equipment to be maintained in the exam room includes the desks, stools, instrument stands, and chairs. A daily dusting is necessary. Cover equipment with an appropriate cover at night. Leave computerized equipment plugged into a surge protector. Some offices choose to unplug certain pieces of equipment at night.

Examination furniture requires very little maintenance. Instrument stands and chairs are designed to provide ease of use, effortless delivery of instruments, and well-balanced, easy to lock instrument arms (Figure 1-2). The slit lamp, phoropter, projector, and keratometer can all be mounted on balanced arms. Many exam chairs have a hydraulic motor that is operated with a foot switch, so that the patient can be positioned properly for various tests. Armrests and footrests can be moved out of the way to help patients move in and out of the chair easily. Some chairs can be tilted back so that the patient is in a supine position for examination with the indirect ophthalmoscope. Some units offer additional outlet switches and room light controls. There may also be a console with charging wells for handheld instruments such as the penlight, retinoscope, and ophthalmoscope. Vinyl upholstery is stain resistant and durable. If the chair will not operate, make sure that the chair/stand unit is plugged in. There is a fuse (usually located in the back of the unit) that may need to be replaced if the unit is not working.

OSHA Standards

Allied health personnel may incur occupational exposure to blood and other potentially infectious material in the eyecare practice. Occupational Safety and Health Administration (OSHA) standards define the need for an exposure plan in the eyecare practice. Some of the tasks performed by ancillary personnel that can expose potentially infectious materials are removing and applying postoperative or post-trauma eye dressings, handling and cleaning instruments, assisting in minor surgical procedures, removal or insertion of contact lenses when corneal disruption or infiltration is present, and any part of an eye exam where bloody discharge is present. Universal precautions can be used to prevent accidental contamination.

Contaminated needles and other contaminated sharps should be placed in a sharps container. Do not recap the needle unless absolutely necessary. Do not bend, break, or shear needles or sharps.

Hand washing is a must in the eyecare practice. Hand washing is one of the most important procedures in the eyecare practice. This should be performed routinely before and after each patient. Disposable gloves should be worn when it is anticipated that there will be contact with blood or any other potentially contaminated or infectious material. Gloves should only be used once and must be replaced as soon as they become contaminated. Change gloves as soon as feasible if they become torn, punctured, or their ability to function as a barrier is compromised. Utility gloves should be worn by housekeeping. These gloves can be reused if they are decontami-

Figure 1-2. Instrument stands and chairs have arms to hold all equipment needed in the eye exam. (Photograph courtesy of Marco Technologies, Inc.)

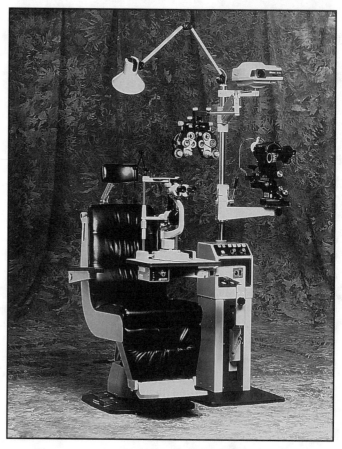

nated, provided that the integrity of the glove is not compromised. Masks and goggles should be used if there is the potential for contaminated sprays or splashes.

Contaminated surfaces should be wiped after the completion of a procedure or as soon as feasible during a procedure. Properly dispose of contaminated material in red boxes. Do not directly handle contaminated material—use tongs or forceps.

It is recommended that eyecare personnel receive the Hepatitis B vaccine if there will be exposure to blood or other potentially infectious material.

HIV in the Eyecare Practice

The risk of acquiring human immunodeficiency virus (HIV) infections during the eye exam is remote. There is a relatively low risk of transmission of the virus through contact with tears. HIV is a very fragile virus. There is no spread from surfaces that do not touch the eye (eg, the slit lamp). The HIV virus can be killed by using an alcohol wipe, 3% hydrogen peroxide, or a solution of 1:10 dilution of household bleach. A tonometer (that touches the eye) should be soaked for at least five minutes then rinsed and dried. A diagnostic contact lens should be disinfected using the same method. Contact lenses used for trial fitting must be disinfected between patients.

Chapter 2

Instruments Used in Determining Visual Acuity

KEY POINTS

- Keep instruments free from dust and fingerprints.
- Change the projector bulb with great care.
- Front surface mirrors must be gently cleaned to protect silver coating.
- Oil and dirt from fingers can damage color vision plates and caps.

The instruments and equipment in this chapter are used in the exam to help determine and measure the visual status of the eye. These instruments are the projector, associated screens and mirrors, distance and near vision charts, the Brightness Acuity Tester, vision screener, color vision plates and tests, the optokinetic drum and tape, and photoscreening devices.

Projectors

Description and Purpose

This instrument (Figure 2-1) is used to project symbols onto a screen to obtain a subjective visual acuity. A slide is inserted into the instrument that has a choice of characters that can be used on adults or children. A vectograph slide is available to be used with polarizing glasses so that each eye can be tested independently. The projector is usually wall mounted or can stand on a table or floor. Some projectors can utilize a long-life halogen bulb that gives a longer service per bulb and provides a brighter whiter light.

Maintenance

As with all equipment used in eyecare, keeping the projector clean and free of dust is one of the most important steps in its maintenance. Cover it at night and when not in use. The body of the projector can be dusted with a soft cloth. Turning the instrument off when not in use will provide longer hours of operation. The life span of the projector bulb is affected by the amount of time the bulb is lit. Heat buildup in the housing and the amount of voltage that passes through the filament can also decrease a bulb's life. To replace a bulb, unplug the unit then open the projector and remove the bulb housing. Do not try to remove a blown bulb until the bulb and its housing are cool. Hold the new bulb using a tissue or a rubber bulb holder. This will protect your hands from cut glass in the event the glass bulb jacket breaks. Also, a tissue or bulb holder will prevent an oily imprint on the bulb jacket that can be etched into the glass and may cause a shadow in the illumination field (Figure 2-2). The bulb may need to be rotated to its full extent if shadows or incomplete illumination occurs on the screen. Sometimes the housing that contains the projector's concave mirror is not in place properly behind the bulb, and may need to be adjusted so that it is directly in line with the bulb. There are small screws that are loosened and the mirror can be shifted to allow for better illumination. (Always make sure the bulb is good before attempting other measures to improve screen illumination.) Check the bulb's contacts when changing the bulb. If corrosion is apparent, it can be scraped off with an eraser or file.

The projector lens can be dusted with canned air. Stubborn dust may be removed with a camel hair brush. A quality lens solution can be used if needed. Slightly dampen a lens wipe and gently clean the lens surface.

Power Supply

A wall socket cord supplies power to the projector. Problems with the projector can be caused by a defective cord, a loose connection, or corroded contacts. If none of the above are a problem, check the outlet itself—wall sockets can be defective. It is important to check the viability of the socket before sending the instrument for service that may not be needed.

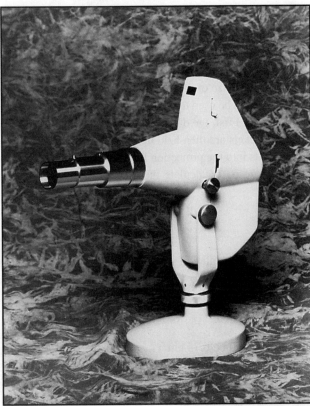

Figure 2-1. Visual acuity projector. (Photograph courtesy of Marco Technologies Inc.)

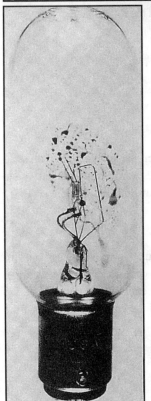

Figure 2-2. A fingerprint etched into a bulb glass jacket. (Reprinted from Blair B, Appleton B, Garber N, Crowe M, and Alven M. *Opticianry, Ocularistry and Ophthalmic Technology.* Thorofare, NJ: SLACK Incorporated; 1990.)

Calibration

The projector has slides that are to be used in a 20 ft examining lane. A 20/20 symbol will subtend an angle of 5 min of arc. At 20 ft this image will be 9 mm high. A 20/200 symbol will be 9 cm tall. However, most examining rooms are not 20 ft in length. The projector has a projection tube that, when moved in and out, changes the size of the symbols. The manual that accompanies the projector has projection brackets that can be used to obtain proper image size when the distance from the patient to the chart is not 20 ft. First, the distance between the patient and the chart is carefully measured. The projection brackets are then held up on the screen and the tube is moved in and out until the 20/200 symbol fits into the projection bracket. (Figure 2-3).

Another method of determining symbol size is to calculate the appropriate symbol height using the following formula:

$$\frac{\text{the size of symbol needed (x)}}{\text{9cm (20/200 @ 20 ft)}} = \frac{\text{patient distance}}{\text{20 ft}}$$

If the patient is 15 ft away from the screen the calculation would be:

$$\frac{\text{the size of symbol needed (x)}}{\text{9 cm}} = \frac{\text{15 ft}}{\text{20 ft}}$$

$$\text{(x)} = 6.75 \text{ cm}$$

The required height of the 20/200 symbol would be 6.75 cm.

In many short eyecare exam rooms, mirrors are used to obtain a 20 ft test distance. Front surface mirrors are used because they reflect 100% of the transmitted light. Two front surface mirrors and a screen are needed to obtain proper image size. The room length is measured and this distance is added to the patient's distance from the viewing mirror. This total distance must measure 20 ft (Figure 2-4).

Projector Slides

Description and Purpose

The slides (Figure 2-5) that are used in projectors are usually interchangeable among all standard projectors. The slides can easily be changed quickly during the exam. Adult, pediatric, and vectograph (used to determine stereopsis in the distance) slides are available.

Maintenance

The slides that are used in the projector must be handled carefully to prevent dust and fingerprints. To remove fingerprints, carefully wipe the glass surfaces with a clean, dry lens wipe. Never place the slide under running water or spray solutions on it, because it is composed of two glass plates with the acuity symbols between them. Water or solutions can seep inbetween the glass and ruin or distort the symbols.

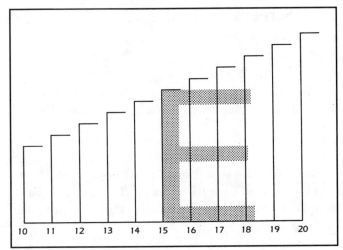

Figure 2-3. Brackets (not to scale) used to calibrate the 20/200 symbol for the correct visual angle for 20/- notation. (Reprinted from Blair B, Appleton B, Garber N, Crowe M, and Alven M. *Opticianry, Ocularistry and Ophthalmic Technology.* Thorofare, NJ: SLACK Incorporated; 1990.)

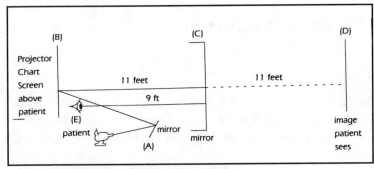

Figure 2-4. Set up for projecting a 20/20 visual angle symbol using front surface mirrors in a room less than 20 feet. (Reprinted from Blair B, Appleton B, Garber N, Crowe M, and Alven M. *Opticianry, Ocularistry and Ophthalmic Technology.* Thorofare, NJ: SLACK Incorporated; 1990.)

Figure 2-5. Slides used in projectors showing various symbols.

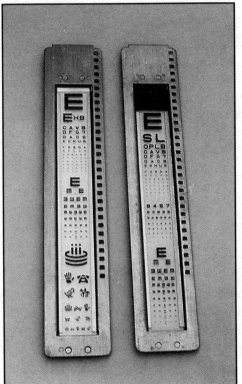

Screens

Description and Purpose

Screens (Figure 2-6) are used to reflect the light and symbols from a projector. A top quality screen should be used so that the projected light is transmitted off of it as much as possible.

Maintenance

Although most of the screens available today are washable, great care is still needed when cleaning, because frequent wiping and washing will erode the screen's surface over a period of time. The screen should never be touched with fingers or sharp instruments. Clean the screen with a mild soap solution if it is a washable type.

 # Front Surface Mirrors

Description and Purpose

Mirrors are used in exam rooms that are not 20 ft long. A longer refracting lane can be obtained when two front surface mirrors are used. Front surface mirrors (see Figure 2-6) have a coating of silver on the top of the glass. The projected light is bounced off the front surface to produce 100% light transmission.

Maintenance

Great care must be used to maintain this piece of equipment. The silver coating can be easily scratched or removed with improper cleaning. Clean the mirrors only when absolutely necessary and using proper techniques. (Never leave this job to the cleaning crew at night!) The first step in cleaning the mirrors is to remove dust particles with canned air, an ear bulb, or a camel hair brush. Stubborn stains or fingerprint oils can be removed by dragging a slightly damp lens wipe moistened with four parts ether to one part water. Remember this will clean the mirror's surface, but with each cleaning a small amount of silver is removed.

 # Distance and Near Vision Charts

Description and Purpose

Vision charts (Figure 2-7) are used for measuring visual acuity. Standardized optotypes are used. Most charts available today are printed on laminated cardboard or plastic. Distance charts are available for both 10 and 20 ft distances. Near visual acuity charts are designed to be tested at 16 inches. Most cards are also printed on plastic surfaces.

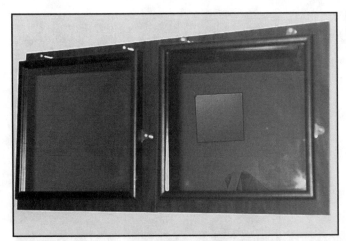

Figure 2-6. A screen is reflected in the front surface mirror.

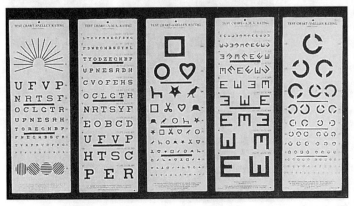

Figure 2-7. Distance visual acuity charts. (Reprinted from Herrin MP. *Ophthalmic Examination and Basic Skills.* Thorofare, NJ: SLACK Incorporated; 1990.)

Maintenance

Charts printed on plastic surfaces can easily be washed with a mild soap solution. Cardboard charts that are not laminated will soil easily when touched. Oils and dirt from fingers can ruin the charts.

Brightness Acuity Tester (BAT)

Description and Purpose

The Brightness Acuity Tester (Figure 2-8) provides objective measurements of functional visual acuity in different light conditions. Cataracts can scatter light, causing glare and impaired visual function in bright light conditions. The BAT simulates bright overhead sunlight, indirect sunlight, and bright overhead fluorescent lighting.

Maintenance

The BAT is a hand-held instrument that has a white hemispherical reflector which can become soiled or scratched. The reflector can be removed for cleaning by taking out the retaining screw below the reflector on the front of the instrument. The reflector will then slide down

Figure 2-8. Brightness Acuity Tester (BAT). (Photograph courtesy of Marco Technologies Inc.)

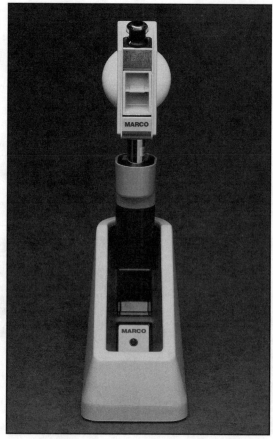

and out. It can be washed with a mild nonabrasive soap or detergent that does not contain lanolin or hand lotion. (The matte surface can absorb such oils.) Dry by gently patting the surface with a lint-free cloth, or allow it to air dry. Do not vigorously rub the matte surface. The reflector should be replaced if the above procedure does not sufficiently clean the surface. The reflector is placed back on the instrument by sliding the notch at the top behind the lamp shield while positioning the circular opening around the lamp. The retaining screw is set into place and tightened only after the center of the reflector aligns perfectly with the aperture in the housing.

It is recommended that the bulb be changed after approximately 15 hours of use on the high setting. The bulb is replaced by removing the cap at the top of the BAT; the bulb will fall out by inverting the instrument. A new bulb is slid into place. Do not touch the glass jacket of the bulb as fingerprint oils can etch into the glass. Replace the locking screw.

Power Supply

The BAT has a rechargeable battery pack and its own charging stand. Do not place the BAT in other charging wells. Once fully charged, the BAT can operate for approximately 30 minutes. If the battery is fully depleted, a full charge can be achieved in 2 hours. The battery can be replaced by unscrewing the end cap from the BAT handle base, and the old battery will slide out. Place it in the charger overnight to ensure full charge of the new battery.

Vision Screener

Description and Purpose

The vision screener (Figure 2-9) is a portable screening system for measuring visual acuity without the use of wall or near vision charts. Acuity can be measured at distance and near, right eye, left eye, or both eyes together. Some machines can determine phorias, evaluate color vision, and measure depth perception. Test slides can be changed for adult or pediatric characters. Some vision screeners have perimetric capabilities. Vision screeners are most commonly seen in schools, drivers license facilities, and military institutions.

Maintenance

Covering the vision screeners will keep the instrument clean and free of dust, and reduce the number of times the test slides and viewing lenses must be cleaned. Over time the test slides must be cleaned. Inside the access there is a drum that contains all the slides. The drum is rotated (usually by pressing the advance pad) and each slide is removed and cleaned with a lens tissue or a lens cleaning towelette. The viewing lenses must be cleaned more often because they are exposed to the patients. Use a lens wipe to clean viewing lenses.

Most vision screener use two lamps for illumination. Change both bulbs when one is burned out to achieve a more consistent illumination. The bulbs are located by removing the top cover and identifying the bulb housing. The lamp housing can be gently lifted out, once the fasteners are removed. Most lamps are of the push/pull type.

The vision screener perimeter lamps must also be changed. Remove the plate on the front of the screener to expose the perimeter lamps and give the bulb a one-quarter turn. (They are not of the push/pull type like the illumination bulbs.)

Power Supply

If the instrument fails to turn on, make sure that the screener is plugged in. Test the wall outlet to make sure it is working properly. If there is still no power, a fuse may need to be changed. The fuse is usually located next to the plug at the rear of the machine. The fuse holder can be pried out gently with a screwdriver; the fuse is replaced with a 2 amp 5x20 fast acting fuse. Gently push the fuse holder back in. Send the machine to the manufacturer if the above steps fail to restore proper working order.

HRR Color Blindness Plates and Ishihara Color Deficiency Test Books

Description and Purpose

These test books (Figure 2-10) are used to determine color blindness. They contain plates to quickly determine blue/yellow and red/green color deficiencies. They further separate the anomaly into mild, medium, or strong color deficiencies. The patient flips through the album of colored plates and is asked to determine the shapes or numbers present.

Figure 2-9. Titmus 2a vision screener. (Photograph courtesy of Titmus Optical, Inc.)

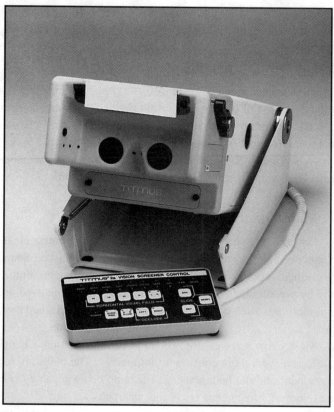

Maintenance

It is important to instruct the patient to identify the shapes on the plates verbally without actually touching the plates. Oils and dirt from fingers can soil the plates over time if patients are repeatedly allowed to trace around the shapes with their fingers.

Farnsworth Dichotomous 15 and 100 Hue

Description and Purpose

These color vision tests contain 15 or 100 colored caps, respectively, that are used to determine color vision anomalies (Figure 2-11a, b). The patient places the caps in order of color progression. The caps have numbers printed on the bottoms of them. After the patient has finished the test, the caps are flipped over and the numbers are charted (in the order that they were placed) on score sheets.

Maintenance

Advise the patient not to touch the colors on the caps. Oils and dirt from fingers can easily soil colors on caps, changing their hue and/or intensity.

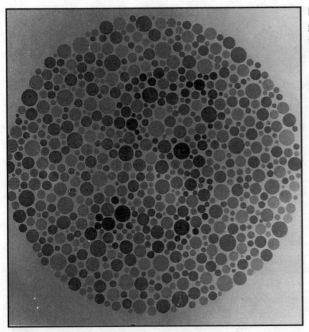

Figure 2-10. Black and white photograph of a test plate from Ishihara's Test for Colour-Deficiency, Kanehara & Co. Ltd.

Optokinetic Drum and Tape

Description and Purpose

The optokinetic (OKN) drum (Figure 2-12a) is used to determine the presence of visual acuity. The drum is rotated in front of a patient and the patient's eye will move in the direction of the drum rotation. There are two types of drums, one is striped and the other has children's pictures on it. The drum rotates on a ball bearing system.

The optokinetic tape (Figure 2-12b) is a cloth tape with squares sewn on it. It is also used to determine presence of visual acuity. The tape is moved in front of the patient's eyes. The eyes will naturally move in the direction of the tape movement.

Maintenance

Little maintenance is required on the optokinetic drum. It rotates on a ball bearing system and can be wiped clean with a mild soap solution if needed.

Photoscreening Devices

Purpose and Description

Photoscreening devices use a Polaroid™ camera with special film to take an instant picture of a preschool child's eyes. The resultant photo of the pupillary reflexes can be evaluated to identify the possible presence of strabismus, refractive errors, opacities, or other abnormalities. This instrument provides an objective assessment on the visual status of non-verbal children's eyes. It

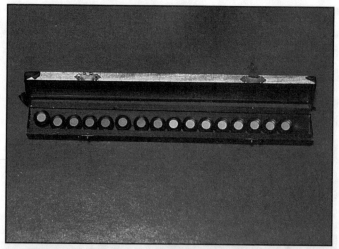

Figure 2-11a. Farnsworth Dichotomus 15 Hue Test. (Photograph by Rhonda Curtis, COT, CRA.)

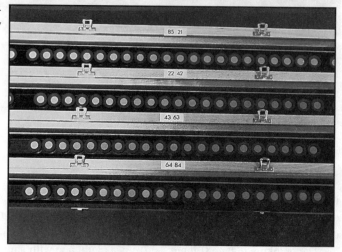

Figure 2-11b. Farnsworth Dichotomus 100 Hue Test. (Photograph by Rhonda Curtis, COT, CRA.)

is very useful in very small and difficult to evaluate children because there is no need for verbal interaction with the child.

Maintenance

The photoscreener should be covered at night and and kept away from any water source. It can be wiped clean with a damp cloth. No solutions or chemicals should be used on the photoscreener. When service or repair work is needed, the instrument should be sent to an authorized service center. No attempt should be made to disassemble the photoscreener. Opening or removing covers could expose one to highly dangerous voltages.

The MTI Photoscreener (Medical Technologies and Innovations Inc) uses MTI 3200 B/W film. The film should be loaded so that the cardboard side is facing up and the yellow pull tab faces outward. Open the film door and gently push the film cartridge into place. Then close the film door until the latch clicks.

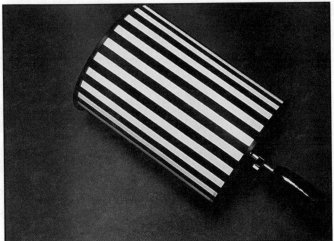

Figure 2-12 a. Optokinetic drum. (Photograph by Rhonda Curtis, COT, CRA.)

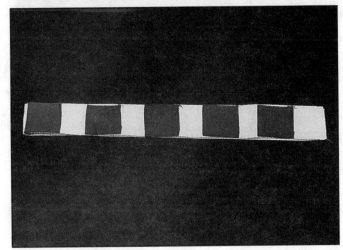

Figure 2-12 b. Optokinetic tape. (Photograph by Rhonda Curtis, COT, CRA.)

The instrument has a rechargeable battery along with an external AC/DC adapter. The rechargeable battery takes 14 hours to charge. As with all rechargeable batteries, the battery's life can be extended if recharging occurs only when the battery is low. (A blinking light indicates a low battery.) The instrument is plugged into the AC/DC adapter and can still be used during the charge period. Do not use the photoscreener during an electrical storm as this can result in an electrical shock.

Chapter 3

Instruments Used to Determine the Refractive State of the Eye

KEY POINTS

- Cover all instruments at night to protect them from dust.

- There are 168 lens surfaces to clean on the phoropter.

- Lenses in the phoropter are protected when the dials are set to zero.

- Turn off the lensmeter when finished; do not leave it on all day.

- Leave the retinoscope out of the charger during daily use to discharge the battery.

The following instruments are used in the eye exam to measure the refractive state of the eye. These instruments are the phoropter, autorefractor, retinoscope, lensmeter, trial frames and lenses, cross cylinder, and distometer.

Phoropter

Description and Purpose

The phoropter is a refracting instrument that was developed over 70 years ago (Figure 3-1). This piece of equipment has made refractometry easy to perform with maximum accuracy because lenses are easily changed in .25 or 3.00 diopter increments. The phoropter is a large, strange looking pair of glasses that contains several internal spherical and cylindrical lenses, and an external rotating turret that carries a cross cylinder and a rotary prism. There are several auxiliary lenses in the phoropter including a retinoscopic lens (automatically removes the examiner's working distance), red or green filter lenses, vertical and horizontal Maddox Rods, a pinhole, dissociating prisms, a fixed cross cylinder, an occluder, and a polarizing analyzer. The phoropter has a detachable reading rod that can be used to determine near vision add or measure amplitudes of accommodation. The Risley prisms can be used to determine both horizontal and vertical fusional amplitudes.

Maintenance

Keeping the phoropter clean and free of dust is one of the most important steps in instrument maintenance. All lenses and auxiliary lenses should be set to zero or open after using the phoropter. This leaves an open aperture and keeps the lenses protected in the body. One should never attempt to determine if the aperture is open by inserting a finger in the opening. This will soil the lenses. One can keep the instrument clean by simply dusting the exterior surface with a soft cloth and covering at night. The face shields attached to the back can be washed with soap and water, soaked in alcohol, or sterilized in an autoclave.

There are several factors around the office that contribute to the amount of lens soilage. One contributing factor may be that the office is located near a factory and windows are often left open, or that smoking is permitted in the office. It is recommended that the phoropter be sent to a trained professional yearly for cleaning and lubricating. If you choose to clean the lenses yourself, read on, but beware that there are 168 lens surfaces to clean!

The lenses can be cleaned without opening the phoropter casing. The lenses are cleaned as they are rotated through the opening. The use of indirect illumination is very useful to help identify soiled lenses. Canned air or a rubber ear syringe can be used to remove dust particles from the lens surfaces by gently blowing on the surface. A camel hair brush can be used on the lens for stubborn debris. Figure 3-2 shows how to make a cleaning tool. The tool can be moistened with a lens cleaning solution. Never spray a cleaner directly into the phoropter—this can be harmful to the phoropter. The lenses should be cleaned in the following order, which allows for all lenses to be cleaned without repetition. Set the phoropter to zero or open and start with the cylindrical lenses in the following order: .25, .50, .75, 1.00, 1.25, 2.50, 3.75, and 5.00. Remember to clean both the front and back surface of each lens from the front and back side of the phoropter.

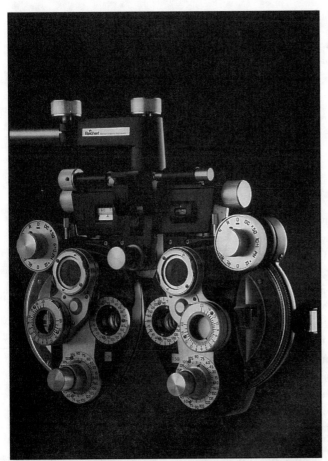

Figure 3-1. Ultramatic RxMaster™ Phoropter®. (Photograph courtesy of Reichert Ophthalmic Instruments, a Division of Leica.)

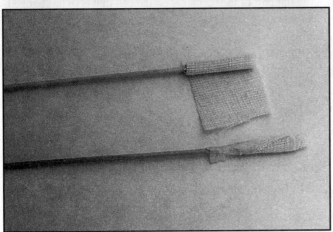

Figure 3-2. Cleaning tool made by rolling a strip of soft, lint-free linen around a cotton swab and secure with tape.

Clean spherical lenses in the following order: +1.75, +1.50, +1.25, +1.00, +.75, +.50, +.25, -.25, -.50, -.75, and -1.00, once again, front and back. Then clean the strong sphere powers (3.00 diopter increments) in the following order: +3.00, +6.00, +9.00, +12.00, +15.00, -18.00, -15.00, -12.00, -9.00, -6.00, and -3.00.

The auxiliary lenses are cleaned next, followed by those in the rotating turrets. Clean the front and back surfaces of the cross cylinder and the rotary prism. That was 168 lens surfaces, and you are done!

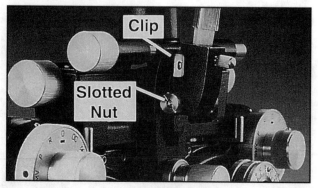

Figure 3-3. Location of slotted nut used to tighten reading rod. (Photograph courtesy of Reichert Ophthalmic Instruments, a Division of Leica.)

The hinged reading rod is held in place by a spring clip and occasionally the tension needs to be tightened. Two screwdrivers are needed—place one screwdriver in the slotted nut and the other in the slotted nut on the other side. Gently tighten the nut. The reading rod slips into place by a bearing which can sometimes require lubrication. Place a drop or two of oil into the oil hole near this bearing when needed. Figure 3-3 shows the location of the slotted nut.

The tension of the cylinder, sphere, and auxiliary dials can easily be adjusted by using a 5/64 Allen wrench. The lenses are on rolling index wheels. The lens wheel should rotate freely without sticking while providing enough tension to prevent lenses from slipping. The adjusting screws (Figure 3-4) are located on the bottom of the phoropter. To tighten tension rotate the wrench in a clockwise manner. To decrease tension, rotate the wrench in a counterclockwise direction. This adjustment must be performed individually for each of the three dials.

Occasionally different lenses are needed in the auxiliary dial. These can easily be replaced using a screwdriver. The auxiliary dial is rotated until one of the two screws that holds the lens to be changed is visible in the rear of the main aperture. (Figure 3-5.) Loosen the screw without removing, and rotate the washer until the flat part of the washer is on the cell that is to be changed. Re-tighten the screw. The auxiliary dial is rotated until the other screw that holds the lens cell is visible— repeat the same step by rotating the washer. The auxiliary lens dial is rotated so that the lens cell is in the center of the aperture. Gently press the lens out of the auxiliary dial through the rear aperture and replace it with the new lens. Lock the lens by rotating the washers and tightening the screws.

Autorefractor

Description and Purpose

The autorefractor (Figure 3-6) is a precision optical instrument that can automatically determine refractive measurements of the eye. Some instruments have a chin rest, forehead rest, and viewing screen for the observer to monitor fixation. The Nidek RT-2100 resembles a phoropter with a combined chart projector, a control box, and printer. It will measure the refractive error, balance both eyes, determine the presence of a phoria and its amount, perform a Worth 4 Dot, measure the Near Point of Accomodation (NPA), and Near Point of Convergence (NPC).

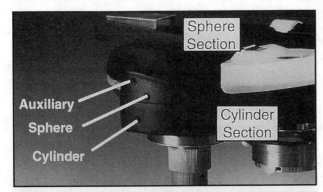

Figure 3-4. Location of adjusting screws on phoropter. (Photograph courtesy of Reichert Ophthalmic Instruments, a Division of Leica.)

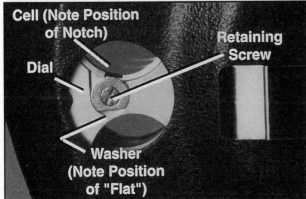

Figure 3-5. Auxilliary dial removable cell viewed through the rear of main aperture. (Photograph courtesy of Reichert Ophthalmic Instruments, a Division of Leica.)

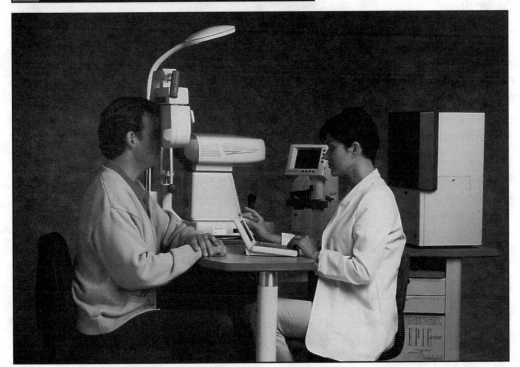

Figure 3-6. Nidek RT-2100 Auto Refractor. (Photograph courtesy of Marco Technologies, Inc.)

Maintenance

There is little maintenance on an autorefractor because this instrument is basically a computer. It has high voltage electronic parts inside; therefore, one should never attempt to disassemble or touch the inside of this instrument. It should be maintained in the same way you would maintain a computer. Always cover the autorefractor at night to keep dust and debris off of the instrument. The forehead rest, chin rest, and face shields should be cleaned with an alcohol wipe between patients. Some instruments have chin rest papers that can be used. Never spray harsh cleaners directly on the instrument.

Maintenance for the Nidek RT-2100 will be described. Refer to the manual for other instrument types. The measuring window can become dusty or soiled by smudges from the patient's nose, lashes, or fingers. These smudges may affect the accuracy of the refraction. Gently use an ear syringe bulb to blow dust from the window's surface. Use a lens wipe to remove nose or fingerprint oils. Do not touch the measuring window with your fingers and advise the patient not to touch this surface. Always make sure that the refractor head is fixed securely. If it drops there is a possibility of injury or damage.

The instrument prints the results on paper that have a red marking to indicate when the roll is nearing its end. The roll of paper can easily be removed. Push the printer part once and slide it out. The shaft is removed from the paper core and a new roll is inserted and is fed into the paper inlet. The paper will feed through the printer as the gear is turned. The results are thermally printed, so make sure to insert the new roll in the proper position so that the results are printed on the correct side.

Power Supply

The autorefractor uses a power cord that attaches to the unit and a wall socket. If the instrument does not operate and the wall socket is working, check the fuses in the instrument. Always turn the instrument off and disconnect the power supply from the wall outlet before attempting to replace the fuses. The fuse plug should be gently removed and the fuses replaced with the type recommended by the manufacturer.

Calibration

Model eyes are used to check that the instrument is in proper working condition. Because these instruments are computers, an error message will often be given by the machine if there is a malfunction.

Streak or Spot Retinoscope

Description and Purpose

The streak or spot retinoscope (Figure 3-7) is a hand-held instrument that is used to objectively determine the refractive power of the eye. A streak or spot of light is reflected off of a front surface mirror. This light is emitted from the instrument and the streak type can be rotated 360 degrees. The retinoscope comes in two types—a standard and a halogen. The halogen model gives a brighter and whiter light source.

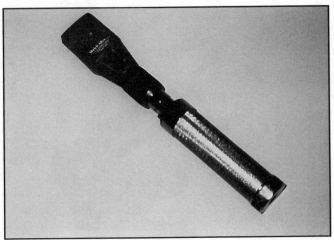

Figure 3-7. Welch Allyn Retinoscope.

Maintenance

The retinoscope has a bulb, a front surface mirror to reflect the light, and a battery or transformer. The Copeland 180 degree Streak Retinoscope has a push-and-pull type lamp. The thumb slide is pulled out and the retinoscope head slides out to expose the bulb. Do not try to turn or twist the bulb while changing it, as this will ruin the base. The Welch Allyn has a bulb that slides into the head when the head has been removed from the battery base. The old bulb is easily removed by gently flipping it out with a screwdriver. It is important to know which type of bulb the retinoscope uses. Bulbs can easily be damaged if not inserted or removed properly. The retinoscope should be turned off immediately after use. The bulb can get extremely hot during use and the filament can bend if the instrument is left on its side while turned on. This creates a C-shape in the filament and can affect the light emitted from the retinoscope.

Power Supply

The retinoscope can have a cord, a self-contained power supply (rechargeable handle), or it may be attached to a transformer. The retinoscope is sensitive to high voltages, and bulbs will blow if a transformer is left at a too high setting.

Lensmeter

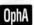

Description and Purpose

The lensmeter (Figure 3-8) is an instrument used to measure the spherical and cylindrical power and the axis of the cylinder in a spectacle or contact lens. The presence of prism and the direction of its base can also be determined using the lensmeter. The instrument consists of an eyepiece, a stage on which to set the spectacles or contact lens, a power wheel, and an illumination source. Most instruments also have a lens marking device. The dioptric range of some instruments can go to plus or minus 30 diopters. There are two types of targets that are used in these instruments. The American or Cross-Line target incorporates one line crossed by three lines, and the Corona Dot target uses a series of dots in a circle.

Figure 3-8. Lensmeter. (Photograph courtesy of Marco Technologies, Inc.)

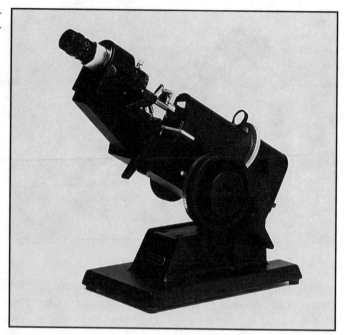

Maintenance

The lensmeter uses an eyepiece that must be focused for each individual user. This lens can be kept clean by covering the instrument at night. Canned air or a camel hair brush can be used to remove any dust. The eyepiece can be wiped with a lens wipe if smudges or mascara soil the lens. Lensmeter bulbs have a long life. However, the lensmeter should still be turned off between use. The Marco lensmeter has a lamp housing with a hinged cover that is flipped open; the bulb is removed and a new one is screwed into place. Refer to your user's manual for other manufacturer's brands. Check contact points when changing the bulb. Most lensmeters have a marking device. To change the ink pad, slide the pad out and insert a new one. The marking pens should be cleaned periodically with an alcohol wipe to prevent ink buildup.

Power Supply

Lensmeters may use standard batteries or electricity. Check the cord and wall socket if the electric lensmeter does not function.

Calibration

The eyepiece is set for the examiner before use. Standard trial lenses are used to determine the accuracy of the lensmeter. Power discrepancy may be found when testing extremely high powered lenses in the trial lens set. The lensmeter must be returned to the factory if unable to obtain proper readings.

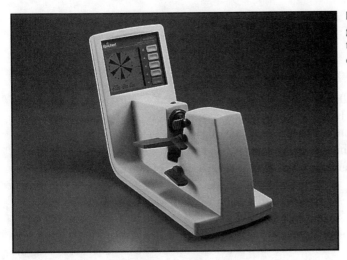

Figure 3-9. LensChek™. (Photograph courtesy of Reichert Ophthalmic Instruments, a Division of Leica.)

Automatic Lensmeter

Description and Purpose

The automatic lensmeter (Figure 3-9) is an easy instrument to use to obtain objective spectacle measurements. The operator need only to insert the spectacles and press appropriate buttons. Spectacles are read automatically, both distance and near. This objective measurement can be important especially when reading progressive addition lenses. The automatic lensmeter uses computer technology.

Maintenance

The automatic lensmeter should be covered at night to prevent build up of dust and debris. The instrument can be wiped with a damp cloth. It is a microprocessor-based instrument. Never use a cleaning spray on the instrument because the solution could get into the machine. As with the manual lensmeter, the ink pad can be slid out and replaced with a new one. The ink pen tips should be wiped periodically to remove any ink build up. The nosepiece cover (the spectacle lens rests against this piece while reading) can become torn or abraded over time and may occasionally need to be replaced. The old cover can be gently pried loose with a screwdriver, and a new piece is attached and then reversed around the unit.

Power Supply

The automatic lensmeter uses a power cord and wall outlet. There are also fuses that may need to be changed in the unit. The LensChek™ by Reichert must be unplugged first from the wall socket and then from the unit itself when changing the fuse.

Trial Frame

Description and Purpose

The trial frame (Figure 3-10) is an adjustable frame that is used with trial lenses when measuring the patient for spectacle lenses. The trial frame accommodates both spherical and cylindrical lenses. The pupillary distance, lens height, cylinder axis, temple length, and inclination can be set to accommodate all patient sizes. Most temples are spring loaded with an adjustable nose rest for patient comfort. Trial frames are lightweight, and made of plastic and metal.

Maintenance

There is little maintenance required for the trial frame. It should be kept clean, and the nose rest should be wiped with an alcohol wipe between patients. Care should be taken not to drop the frame because a hard shock can easily knock the frame out of alignment. The trial frame can be wiped with a soft cloth to keep it free from dust and debris.

Trial Lenses

Description and Purpose

Trial lens sets (Figure 3-11) are a set of lenses used to measure the refractive state of the eye. Trial lenses can be rimmed or rimless.

Maintenance

Trial lenses are most often made of glass. The lenses should be kept in a drawer or covered to keep them clean and dust free. The lenses can be cleaned with a glass cleaner and a soft cotton cloth.

Cross Cylinder

Description and Purpose

The cross cylinder, or Jackson cross cylinder (Figure 3-12), is a compound lens having a net minus power in one principle meridian and a net plus power in the other. The minus axes are marked with a red dot and the plus axes are marked with a white dot. Common powers used in the eye care practice are 0.25, 0.50, and 1.00. The cross cylinder is mounted in a metal frame with a handle that straddles the two principle axis. The cross cylinder can also be mounted to the phoropter. The cross cylinder is used to refine the axis and power of the cylinder when performing refractometry.

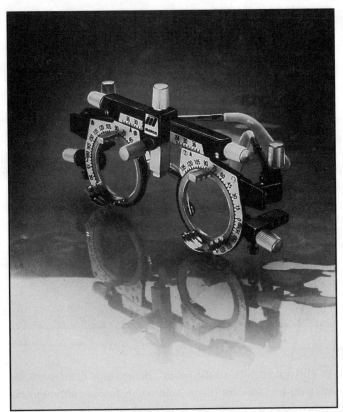

Figure 3-10. Marco trial frame. (Photograph courtesy of Marco Technologies, Inc.)

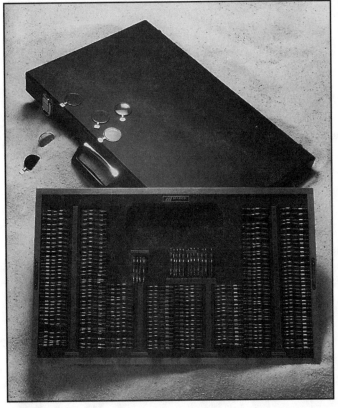

Figure 3-11. Marco trial lens set. (Photograph courtesy of Marco Technologies, Inc.)

Figure 3-12. Jackson cross cylinder.

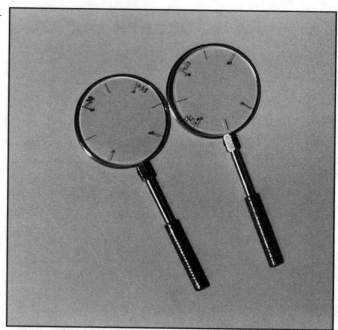

Maintenance

Most cross cylinders are made of glass and can be washed with a damp cloth. Care should be taken not to use harsh detergents when cleaning so that the red and white dots are not removed. Also, the lens should not be rubbed so vigorously that it is loosened and rotated in the rim.

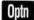

Distometer

Description and Purpose

The distometer (Figure 3-13) is an important instrument used in measuring vertex distance, the distance between the phoropter or trial lens surface and the eye. This distance is crucial when prescribing high lens refractions. A circular conversion chart enables the prescriber to convert the prescription taking the vertex distance into account.

Maintenance

The distometer should be kept in a drawer. Care should be taken to prevent dropping the instrument on a hard surface. A hard shock to the instrument can damage it and change the reading.

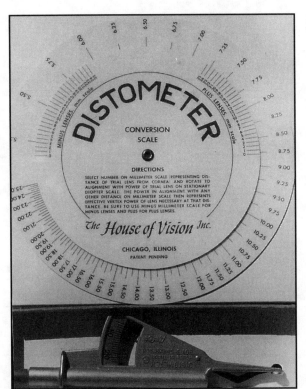

Figure 3-13. Distometer by House of Vision.

Chapter 4

Instruments Used to Evaluate Ocular Motility and Determine the Binocular Status of the Eye

- Place instruments in carrying cases or in a drawer when not in use.

- Never use alcohol on plastic prisms.

- Dry or polish prisms with soft cotton cloths to prevent scratches.

- Advise patients not to touch circles or animals on the stereo test.

- Remove batteries from the Worth 4 Dot if not used on a regular basis.

The following instruments are used to determine ocular motility and the status of binocular vision. These instruments are loose prisms, prism bar, Risley prism, stereopsis tests, the Maddox Rod, the Worth 4 Dot, and Bagolini lenses.

Loose Prisms

Description and Purpose

A prism (Figure 4-1) is a triangular piece of glass or plastic that has flat sides with an apex and a base. Prisms bend light rays, and when placed in front of the eye can be used with appropriate tests to measure a phoria or a tropia. Loose prisms come in sets of 16 or 22.

Maintenance

Keep prisms in the carrying case. This will keep the prisms clean and dust free. Prisms that are made of glass can be cleaned with any solution that may be used on glass. Most prisms available today are acrylic or lucite which should not be exposed to solutions (including alcohol) that can alter the surface. Alcohol can cause the surface of the prism to become white and foggy. When cleaning the prisms care should be taken not to scratch the plastic surface. Special soft cotton cloths can be used on the plastic surfaces that will not scratch them.

Prism Bar

Description and Purpose

The prism bar (Figure 4-2) has plastic prisms that are attached to each other. The prisms in the horizontal bar are 1, 2, 4, 6, 8, 10, 12, 14, 16, 18, 20, 25, 30, 40, and 45 prism diopters. The horizontal prism bar is used for measuring phorias and tropias and for measuring fusional amplitudes (both convergence and divergence). The vertical prism bar has prisms with 1, 2, 3, 4, 5, 6, 8, 10, 12, 14, 16, 18, 20, and 25 prism diopters. The vertical bar is used to measure hyperphorias or hypertropias, or can be used to measure vertical amplitudes.

Maintenance

The maintenance of the prism bars is the same as maintenance for loose prisms. A leather carrying case is usually provided with the prism bar.

Rotary or Risley Prism

Description and Purpose

The rotary or Risley prism is one prism set into a casing that can be rotated to change the amount of prism diopter power. It can be attached to the phoropter (see Figure 3-1) or is attached to a handle for hand-held use.

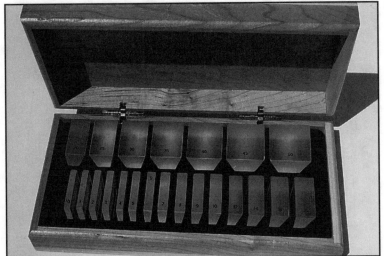

Figure 4-1. Prism set.

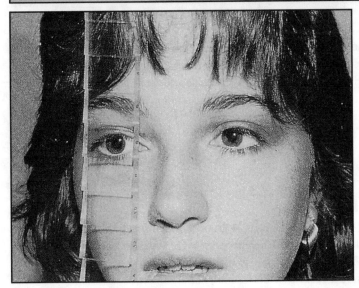

Figure 4-2. Measuring amplitudes of accomodation using prism bar. (Reprinted from Hansen VC. *Ocular Motility.* Thorofare, NJ: SLACK Incorporated; 1986.)

Maintenance

The prism can be cleaned with the same solutions as loose prisms and dried with the same special cloths. Care should be taken that the prism is not immersed into a solution because this can damage the prism carrier and its seal.

Stereopsis Tests

Description and Purpose

The stereoacuity tests (Figure 4-3) utilize a test booklet and polarized glasses to measure stereopsis and depth perception. They measure both gross and fine stereoacuity. The stereo fly test has a house fly for gross stereopsis, an animal selection test for children, and a circle test for older children and adults.

Figure 4-3. Stereo fly test and polarized glasses.

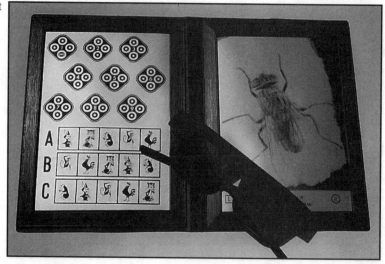

Maintenance

Often the examiner asks the patient to "push the circle in" or to "push the animal in that seems to be off the page or in the air." Constant pushing and touching of circles and animals can damage the test booklet by disrupting the symbols. This may cause a loss of the apparent distance of the objects, falsifying test results. Patients should be asked to point instead.

Maddox Rod

Description and Purpose

The Maddox rod (Figure 4-4) is a series of rods or grooves which function together as a single rod. A light seen through the series of rods appears as a single line. The line appears perpendicular to the axis of the rods. The rod is used to dissociate the eyes. When used with prisms and a light, the examiner can measure a vertical or horizontal phoria.

Maintenance

Clean the Maddox rod as all other hand-held occluders. The plastic carrier can be washed with a mild soap solution or wiped with an alcohol wipe.

Worth 4 Dot

Description and Purpose

The Worth 4 Dot (Figure 4-5) is used to determine visual functions, fusion, suppression, and/or diplopia. The Worth 4 Dot is a flashlight with four dots; the top dot is red, the two side dots are green, and the dot on the bottom is white. Glasses or goggles with one red lens and one green lens are worn by the patient to perform the test.

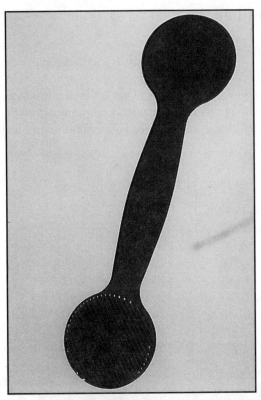

Figure 4-4. Maddox rod.

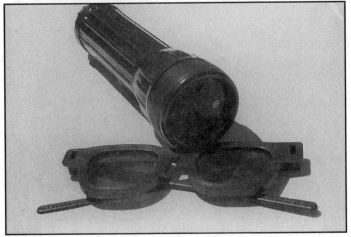

Figure 4-5. Worth 4 Dot flashlight and glasses.

Maintenance

The dots can be kept clean by keeping the flashlight in a drawer and by occasionally dusting off the dots using a cotton swab.

Power Supply

The Worth 4 Dot flashlight operates on standard batteries. Remove the batteries if the flashlight is not used on a regular basis.

Bagolini Lenses

Description and Purpose

Bagolini lenses are finely striated lenses that look like plane glass. They are similar to a Maddox rod. When looking at a light source, the light appears like a fine streak perpendicular to the striation of the lens. The lenses are placed in a trial frame and are used to determine normal and abnormal retinal correspondence.

Maintenance

Bagolini lenses can be cleaned like any glass lens.

Chapter 5

Instruments Used in Determining Intraocular Pressure in the Glaucoma Exam

KEY POINTS

- Proper tonometer calibration is crucial when determining the intraocular pressure.

- Disinfection is important between patients to prevent transfer of infection.

- Never use the Tono-Pen™ XL without the disposable tip cover.

- Always thoroughly dry any probe tip before touching the cornea.

The instruments in this chapter are used in the eye exam to determine intraocular pressure, status of the angle (including trabecular meshwork), and facility of outflow. These instruments include the Schiotz tonometer, applanation tonometer, non-contact tonometers, portable tonometers, Pneumotonometer, and gonioscopy lenses.

Schiotz Tonometer

Description and Purpose

The Schiotz tonometer (Figure 5-1) is a simple, portable, and inexpensive instrument used in the measurement of intraocular pressure (IOP). It is sometimes used in nonophthalmic medical practices, hospitals, and operating rooms. The tonometer consists of a footplate with a central movable plunger that is fitted into a barrel. A weight rests on the plunger, and attached to it is a needle and scale for measurement. The tonometer is placed on the cornea, a reading is taken, and the number is converted to millimeters of Mercury (mm Hg) by using a conversion card.

Maintenance

The Schiotz tonometer must be kept meticulously clean. The plunger must move freely and the footplate must be clean and smooth, without particles. Debris can accumulate in the plunger barrel and on the base of the footplate. Infectious diseases can be transferred between patients if the tonometer is not properly cleaned before each use. The plunger is removed from the barrel and cleaned with alcohol, or both parts can be soaked in 3% hydrogen peroxide. A pipe cleaner works well to clean the inside of the barrel. It is imperative that both parts of the tonometer are completely dry before a pressure measurement is taken. Disposable tonometer covers are available for use to prevent infection transmission from one patient to the next. These covers are convenient since the tonometer will not then have to be cleaned between patients. The tonometer can also be heat sterilized without any damage to the instrument. The testplate used in calibration should also be wiped with alcohol and allowed to dry completely.

Calibration

The tonometer's calibration should be tested before each patient. A test block is provided with each tonometer. The tonometer is help perpendicular to the test block, and when placed on the block the needle should align at the zero position. Failure to hold the instrument properly can result in an error in the reading (Figure 5-2). There is a nut screw on some tonometers that can be loosened so that the needle can be set back to zero. The manual should be consulted before any adjustment is made. Never bend the needle to scale the instrument to zero, as this would produce erroneous measurements. Adding or subtracting from the reading to allow for needle misalignment is also incorrect.

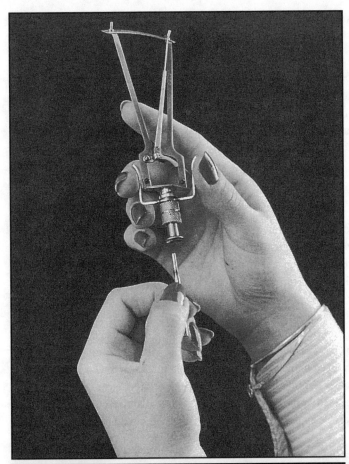

Figure 5-1. Schiotz tonometer with plunger removed for cleaning. (Reprinted from Herrin MP. *Ophthalmic Examination and Basic Skills.* Thorofare, NJ: SLACK Incorporated; 1990.)

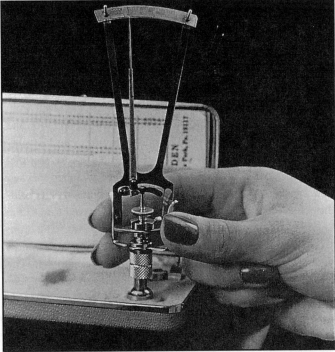

Figure 5-2. Place the tonometer on the test block to test calibration. (Reprinted from Herrin MP. *Ophthalmic Examination and Basic Skills.* Thorofare, NJ: SLACK Incorporated; 1990.)

Applanation Tonometer

Description and Purpose

The Goldmann applanation tonometer (Figure 5-3) is an accurate instrument used in the measurement of IOP. The applanation tonometer measures the force that is required to flatten the cornea in mm Hg. The tonometer tip contacts the eye. A topical anesthetic and fluorescein dye is instilled before measurement of the IOP. The tonometer is used in conjunction with a slit lamp and a cobalt blue filter.

Maintenance

The applanation tonometer requires little maintenance. The applanator head is attached to the tonometer by a pressure sensitive arm. This arm is very delicate and can be easily bent or damaged. The tonometer should never be dropped. The applanator head is a plastic prism that must be cleaned between patients. Failure to clean the head can pass infectious diseases from patient to patient. The head can be soaked for ten minutes in 3% hydrogen peroxide, one part household bleach to ten parts water, or a similar disinfectant that will not damage the plastic prism. After disinfection the prism should be rinsed and dried with a cotton ball. The applanator head should be placed in a suitable container (Petri or other small plastic dish). The applanating surface and 2-3mm of the head should be immersed in the solution. The etching marks on the prism will eventually bleach out if the entire head is left in a solution over a long period of time.

Two applanator heads can be used in one exam room so that one disinfected head is always ready for use. The slit lamp to which the applanation tonometer is attached should be covered at night.

Calibration

Calibration of the applanation tonometer should be performed on a regular basis. There are two models. The 900 series mounts on the Haag-Streit or similar type slit lamp, and the 870 mounts on the tower top of a Humphrey/Zeiss or similar type. First, the measuring prism is put in place. The calibration bar is then attached to the 870 tonometer at the junction of the balance arm (or in the key slot at the side of the 900 model, Figure 5-4) and calibration accuracy is check at drum positions 0 (zero), 2, and 6. The weighted calibration bar has five circles engraved on it. The middle circle corresponds to 0, the two circles next to the middle circle correspond to 2, and the outer circles correspond to 6 on the measuring drum. The 0 (middle circle) is checked first. The weighted bar is aligned at the center circle. The drum is rotated and the pressure arm that holds the tonometer head should be tripped between -.05 and +.05. The tonometer is then checked at position 2. The weighted bar is now moved so that the circle at position 2 is centered in its holder and the longer part of the weight points towards the examiner. (The rod is moved toward the patient when calibrating the 870 and away from the patient when calibrating the 900.) The drum is rotated again and should trip the pressure arm between 1.95 and 2.05. This is the most important position to check because intraocular pressure readings around 20 are very important. The tonometer is then checked again at position 6. The drum is rotated and should trip between 5.95 and 6.05.

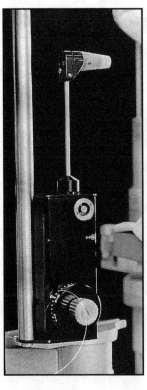

Figure 5-3. Goldmann applanation tonometer attached to the slit lamp. (Reprinted from Herrin MP. *Ophthalmic Examination and Basic Skills.* Thorofare, NJ: SLACK Incorporated; 1990.)

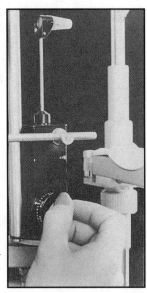

Figure 5-4. Testing the calibration of the Goldmann applanation tonometer with rod. (Reprinted from Herrin MP. *Ophthalmic Examination and Basic Skills.* Thorofare, NJ: SLACK Incorporated; 1990.)

Repair

A tonometer that does not calibrate properly should be sent back to the factory to be repaired. The 870 model can loosen from the tower, throwing alignment off. A screw is located on the back of the plate to adjust the alignment while looking through the left ocular of the slit lamp.

Non-Contact Tonometer (NCT)

Description and Purpose

Non-contact tonometers (Figure 5-5) obtain an objective IOP and do not touch the eye. No anesthesia is required. Some models have a video monitor or a viewing ocular to observe the eye and set up proper alignment. The instrument can be table mounted or hand-held. The readings are taken after a soft and gentle puff of air is directed at the patient's eye. The pressure is displayed on the video monitor or screen readout. Non-contact instruments can be used on almost all patients but is contraindicated in instances of an edematous or ulcerated cornea and following a keratoplasty or penetrating trauma.

Maintenance

There is little maintenance on most non-contact tonometers. A dust cover keeps the instrument dust free overnight and when not in use for a long period of time. It is important to keep the instrument free from dust to eliminate the possibility of a particle from being propelled into a

Figure 5-5. Reichert XPERT™ NCT II™ PLUS. (Photograph courtesy of Reichert Ophthalmic Instruments, a Division of Leica.)

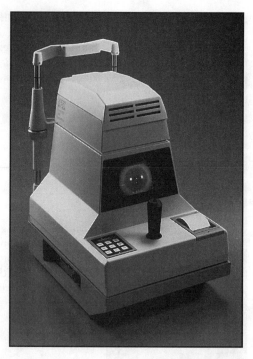

patient's eye by the air pulse. At the start of each day check the air nozzle by firing an air pulse without a patient in place. The fixation area can be cleaned in the case of dust, fingerprints, or eye makeup. A clean, dry cotton swab or a soft, lint-free cotton cloth can be used. The chin cup and forehead rest can be cleaned with an alcohol swab between patients.

Power Supply

A power cord is attached to the instrument and to a working power outlet. Take care to maintain a firm insertion to each. If the instrument does not turn on after the power cord attachments are checked, an internal fuse may have blown and the instrument should be returned for service.

Calibration

Some older models can be calibrated by depressing the trigger switch. Newer models require no calibration and will display "send model for service" if internal calibrations are not attainable.

Portable Tonometers

Portable tonometers allow convenient IOP examinations on hard to examine patients such as children, the elderly, bedside patients, and those in wheelchairs. Several models are available on the market today.

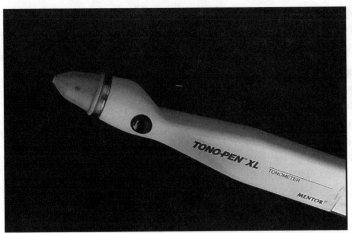

Figure 5-6. Tono-Pen™XL. (Photograph courtesy of Mentor® O&O, Inc.)

Tono-Pen™ XL

Description and Purpose

The Tono-Pen™ XL (Figure 5-6) is a portable instrument used in the measurement of IOP. It is small and lightweight, and it has a self-contained power source. This tonometer looks like a pen. It is lightly touched on an anesthetized cornea which provides a reading in mm of Hg. Disposable tip covers are used to prevent infectious disease transfer between patients.

Maintenance

The Tono-Pen™ XL should be cleaned each day before use. A canister of optical quality gas is needed to maintain this instrument. This gas is used to remove and help prevent buildup around the probe post. This procedure should be done before using each day, before storage at night, and when a good calibration cannot be obtained. The probe tip is inserted into the gas can nozzle. Spray for 2 seconds and wait for 3-4 minutes before checking the instrument's calibration. The Tono-Pen™ XL should be stored in its case at night (not in the lab coat pocket). The batteries should be removed if the tonometer will not be used for an extended period of time.

Power Source

The Tono-Pen™ XL has a self-contained power source. It operates on two 3.0 volt lithium manganese dioxide batteries. Multiple beeps indicate that the batteries in the instrument need to be changed. Replace both batteries by using the stylus blade that accompanies the tonometer. Insert the stylus into the end slot and apply gentle pressure to loosen the battery cover. Insert batteries in the direction shown on the battery compartment floor. Improperly inserted batteries can ruin the tonometer or cause faulty readings. Snap the battery compartment door. Immediately calibrate the tonometer by the following calibration procedure.

Calibration

To calibrate the Tono-Pen™ XL, simply hold the instrument with the tip pointing down at the floor. Then tap the operating button one time, waiting for the word "UP" to appear on the LCD display. Invert the tonometer and point the probe up to the ceiling. The word "GOOD" appears in the display if the calibration was successful.

Perkins Hand-Held Applanation Tonometer

Description and Purpose

The Perkins hand-held applanation tonometer (Figure 5-7) contains the same doubling prism that is used in the slit lamp mounted version. The instrument carries a pair of spiral wound springs that are connected in a series that are tensioned by rotation of the operator's thumb wheel. The resulting force that is stored in the spring is transmitted through the sensitive balanced arm to which the prism is mounted. The measurements can be taken while the patient is seated or supine.

Maintenance

As with the slit lamp mounted version, the pressure sensitive arm should be protected at all times. The prism should be cared for in the same manner as described earlier in this chapter.

Power Supply

The Perkins tonometer uses four standard AA batteries. Two battery-securing buttons are depressed so that the battery case slips away from the instrument. This is the handle portion of the instrument. The batteries must be placed into the compartment as indicated by the symbols in the base.

Repairs

Do not attempt to repair the tonometer. Return it to the factory or supplier for repairs.

Calibration

The calibration of the tonometer should be checked on a regular basis. The batteries must first be removed and the doubling prism is put in place. The thumb wheel is set below zero by the full thickness of one scale line and the prism should tend towards its backward position. Then set the scale reading above zero by the full thickness of one scale line. The prism should then tend towards the forward position of the tonometer. The instrument is then placed on a flat horizontal surface with the setting block under the body near the top (Figure 5-8) and the prism in an upward position. Turn the thumb wheel so that the scale reading is below the 2 mark, by one full thickness of one scale line. A 2 gram weight that comes with the tonometer is placed centrally on the prism and checked to see if it carries the prism positively down to its lowest position. The scale reading is then set above the 2 mark by the full thickness of the scale line and the 2 gram weight is again placed on the prism and checked to see that it remains in its highest position. The above is then repeated at the 5 scale mark using the 5 gram weight that is supplied with the

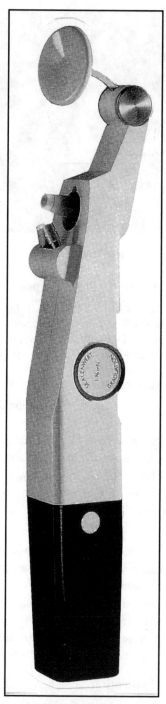

Figure 5-7. Perkins hand-held applanation tonometer. (Photograph courtesy of Haag-Streit.)

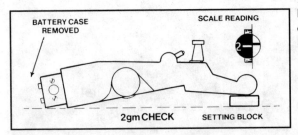

Figure 5-8. Proper placement of tonometer on setting block. (Photograph courtesy of Haag-Streit.)

tonometer. A point of balance can be found at each level. The tolerances at the 0 and 2 gram weights should be + or - .05. At the 5 gram level it should be no more than + or - .075. If the tonometer does not calibrate properly, return the tonometer to supplier.

Pneumotonometer

Description and Purpose

The Pneumotonometer (Figure 5-9) measures IOP through applanation tonometry. A floating pneumatic sensor touches the surface of the anesthetized cornea with the exact amount of force required to take a tonometry or tonographic measurement. The measurements are recorded on a chart. The measurements can be taken while the patient is seated or standing. A tonographic option allows the instrument to obtain a two or four minute tonographic reading. The C value (coefficient of outflow) is automatically calculated and displayed by an internal computer.

Maintenance

The Pneumotonometer should be turned off when not in use. Cover it at night to minimize dust buildup, and dust it periodically with a lint-free cloth. Check the vents on the filter access door for dust.

The thermal paper has a red line along the bottom edge that indicates when the roll is nearing the end. To install a new roll of paper, swing the paper holder out from the console and remove the old roll, taking note of how the paper is fed. The new roll is placed on the spindle counterclockwise. Turn the instrument on so that the "paper feed" option can be used. Feed the paper around the outside roller and in front of the holder, pull three inches out, and close the door. Feed the paper through the inside slot and press the button for paper feed so the paper will advance.

There are two filters on the Pneumotonometer that need to be changed twice a year. Take off the filter access door (on the back) by removing the locking screw at the top. The filter that covers the pump is removed by taking out the anchor screw and replaced with a new filter. The second filter above the pump is held by luer connectors. Rotate the connectors a quarter turn. Remove the old filter and replace with a new filter. Re-install the access cover.

The Pneumotonometer has a probe with a lightweight plastic tip covered by a thin, highly elastic, rubber membrane. The membrane is mounted on a floating piston. The tip must be cleaned after each patient use. The delicate membrane is removed from the tip and the tip is wiped with an isopropyl alcohol pad. The tip must be allowed to dry thoroughly. Inspect the air vents in the tip to make sure that there is no lint in them. Carefully install a new membrane on the tip.

Figure 5-9. Model 30 Classic™ Pneumotonometer. (Photograph courtesy of Mentor® O&O Inc.)

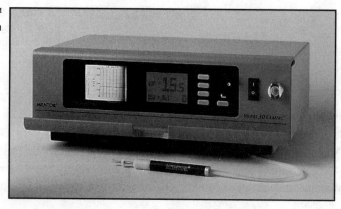

Make sure that the membrane can spin freely. If a second measurement is taken on the same patient, the tip can be wiped with an alcohol pad. Both the tip and membrane can be soaked in alcohol for 10 minutes for a weekly routine cleaning. An inspection with a slit lamp can also help to identify tears, holes, or distortions.

Power Supply

The Pneumotonometer should be turned off when not in use. If the instrument does not function, check the outlet supplying power. There are two fuses below the power cord socket. Replace with time delay fuses, 5x20mm, 1 amp, 250 volt. Pull out the fuse holder and replace any broken or cloudy fuses.

The Goldmann 3 Mirror Lens

Description and Purpose

The Goldmann 3 Mirror Lens (Figure 5-10) is a plastic lens with one or several mirrors inside it. It is used in conjunction with the slit lamp to view the trabecular meshwork and the anterior chamber angle. Following anesthesia, the lens is placed on the eye with a methyl cellulose agent as a buffer fluid and cushion. Once on the eye, the angle and its structures can be easily viewed. Some contact lenses have an attachment that can be used to examine the ora serrata, the pars plana, and most of the peripheral parts of the vitreous and fundus.

Maintenance

Contact glasses are made up of organic glass. It should be cleaned immediately after use. The lens is first washed to remove the cushioning agent and lacrimal fluid. The lens surface can be disinfected in the same manner the applanator heads are cleaned. It is important that the disinfectant does not affect the surface of the plastic, and soaking should only be allowed for 10-20 minutes. Rinse with distilled water and dry with a soft cloth. Do not autoclave or boil the lens. Soaking in alcohol or bleach for a prolonged time would require special care to restrict clouding of the lens and damage to the protective coating or mirrored surface.

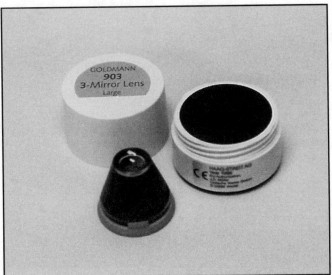

Figure 5-10. The Goldmann 3 Mirror Lens and case by Haag-Streit.

Chapter 6

Instruments Used in Visual Field Testing

KEY POINTS

- Visual fields can aid in detecting glaucoma and neurological disease.

- Instruments must be properly calibrated before use.

- Keep instruments covered at night.

- Automated perimeters are sensitive computerized systems.

The instruments in this chapter are used to determine the visual field. The results of these tests are particularly important in the determination of glaucoma and neurological disease. These instruments are the tangent screen, the Amsler grid, the Goldmann bowl-type perimeter, and the autoperimeter.

Tangent Screen

Description and Purpose

The tangent screen (Figure 6-1) is used to determine the visual field status in the central 30 degrees of the visual field. It is usually made out of black felt. The targets used with the tangent screen are circular disks or balls varying in size and color. A high percentage of field defects are located within the central 30 degrees of the visual field. Therefore, the tangent screen can give excellent information considering its simplicity and affordability.

Maintenance

An occasional whisking with a soft brush to keep dust at a minimum is all the maintenance that is required. A sheet should be placed over the screen at night to help protect it. Tangent screen targets should be kept in a container to keep them clean. Do not touch the target disks or balls, as oils from fingers can soil the targets. These targets can be washed with a mild soapy water if needed. Do not attempt to retouch targets with paint. New targets should be purchased if needed.

Power Supply

There is no power needed to perform this test. However, proper lighting is needed to illuminate the screen. An overhead spotlight aimed at the tangent screen works best. The proper illumination is 7 ft candles.

Calibration

There is no calibration needed on the tangent screen. The test is performed at two distances, 1 and 2 m. These must be carefully measured and kept standard. A piece of tape on the carpet or floor works well.

Amsler Grid

Description and Purpose

The Amsler grid (Figure 6-2) is a chart that was developed to detect small scotomas in the central 20 degrees of the visual field. The chart consists of intersecting lines that form squares that are 5 mm in size. These squares subtend at an angle of 1 degree at 30 cm. The Amsler grid Booklet contains several charts. The chart can have white lines on black paper, or black lines on white. Some charts have red lines, smaller squares that are 1/4 the size of a normal grid, or diagonal lines. A dot is located in the center of the grid for fixation. The Amsler grid is essential in

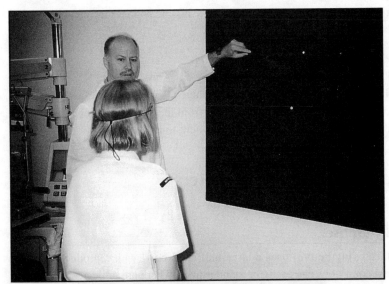

Figure 6-1. Tangent screen. (Reprinted from Choplin N, Edwards R. *Visual Fields.* Thorofare, NJ: SLACK Incorporated; 1998.)

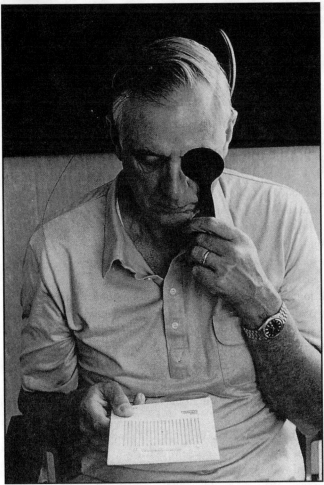

Figure 6-2. Patient using the Amsler grid. (Reprinted from Herrin MP. *Ophthalmic Examination and Basic Skills.* Thorofare, NJ: SLACK Incorporated; 1990.)

following macular degeneration. Pads of Amsler charts are available so that they can be given to adult patients for daily home use.

Maintenance

The booklet should be closed and placed in a drawer when not in use. Care should be taken with the Amsler grid booklet when explaining its use. Soils from the fingers can smudge the central fixation dot if it is touched when showing the patient where to look.

Bowl-Type Perimeters

Description and Purpose

The Goldmann perimeter (Figure 6-3) uses a large half shell bowl with reproducible background lighting so that test conditions can easily be standardized. There are projected test targets of various sizes with several different lighting intensities. The perimeter can quickly test both the peripheral and central visual fields. Patient fixation can be constantly monitored through a viewing device. Some instruments have automatic marking devices.

Maintenance

The perimeter must be covered at night to protect the instrument from dust and debris. The outside of the instrument can be dusted with a soft, lint-free cotton cloth. The inside of the bowl is painted with a special white reflectance paint. Care should be taken NEVER to touch the inside surface of the bowl. When explaining to the patient the fixation target, an over zealous perimetrist will often touch the inside surface. This surface can easily be scratched. To clean the inside surface, first blow dust out of bowl with canned air. Stubborn dust or debris can be removed with a camel hair brush. Extran® MA 02 neutral (Merck) is a product that can be purchased from the manufacturer to clean the inside of the Goldmann. The Extran® is mixed with warm water to make a solution with a concentration of 2%. Use a sponge and rub gently for 5-10 minutes to clean the inside white surface. Rinse the sphere with clear water and a clean sponge, and dry with a soft clean pad. Extran® is biodegradable and nontoxic, and will not irritate the skin.

The projection arm has two ball joints that must have free and smooth movement. To keep this movement smooth, a small drop of thin oil can be used twice a year. Wipe up any excess oil.

The lamp housing (Figure 6-4) should be cleaned with a blast of canned air. The lower surface of the condenser lens collects dust and debris. If it can't be cleaned with the canned air, the lens should be removed and wiped with a soft cloth. To expose the lens, remove the cable for the bulb and press the flanges (on each side of the housing) inwards and the condenser can be removed. Replace the condenser, taking care to properly align the red marks provided for proper placement.

Dirt can collect between the sliding diaphragm and its cylindrical sliding surface on the lamp housing, restricting movement. To remove, pull the diaphragm downward and carefully wipe each surface with a cotton ball moistened with ethyl alcohol. The white plastic foil in the sliding diaphragm becomes loose when removed. When assembling, take care that the white foil lies

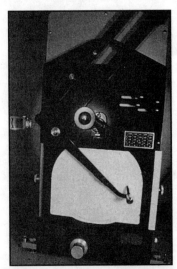

Figure 6-3. Back of the Goldmann perimeter with recording chart in place. (Reprinted from Blair B, Appleton B, Garber N, Crowe M, and Alven M. *Opticianry, Ocularistry and Ophthalmic Technology.* Thorofare, NJ: SLACK Incorporated; 1990.)

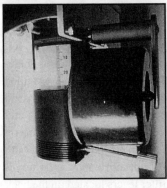

Figure 6-4. Lamp housing of the Goldmann perimeter. (Reprinted from Blair B, Appleton B, Garber N, Crowe M, and Alven M. *Opticianry, Ocularistry and Ophthalmic Technology.* Thorofare, NJ: SLACK Incorporated; 1990.)

exactly between the edges of the diaphragm. Care should be taken not to put too much tension on the diaphragm when returning it onto the cylinder. It can loosen and slip downward, causing a change in the bowl's reflectance.

The machine's bulb is located in the lamp housing at the top of the bowl. The bulb has two sides. This bulb is used to simultaneously illuminate the bowl and project the target. The bulb's life will be extended if it is rotated 180 degrees each week (or after every 20-30 hours of use). If 1000 asb is not achieved during calibration, rotate the bulb to see if the other side has enough illumination. The bulb must be replaced when neither side will achieve 1000 asb. To replace the bulb, turn the machine off and unplug it. Remove the metal plate holding the lamp housing cover in place. The bulb must be rotated and pulled straight out. A new bulb is set in place and rotated to its fullest extent so that the filament will be properly aligned. The housing cover is set back into place and the plate is moved into place to hold the cover. The machine must then be calibrated.

There are two chart illumination bulbs. These lights are located under sliding plates. Remove plates and bulbs to replace.

Power Supply

Make sure that the power cord is attached to a viable outlet. The instrument can be unplugged at night. The fuse holder is located below the light shutter mechanism on the left side of the bowl. If blown, replace with appropriate fuses.

Figure 6-5. To calibrate, move all levers to the right. (Reprinted from Blair B, Appleton B, Garber N, Crowe M, and Alven M. *Opticianry, Ocularistry and Ophthalmic Technology*. Thorofare, NJ: SLACK Incorporated; 1990.)

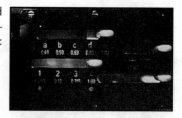

Calibration

The calibration of the perimeter is very important and should be performed on a regular basis. The target illumination is performed first, then the bowl illumination. The target illumination should be rechecked during the day if a large numbers of fields are to be performed. However, the bowl illumination should be calibrated before each patient, with the patient seated in front of the perimeter. This must be done because the color of clothing that the patient is wearing can change the setting for the bowl.

To calibrate the perimeter, the room lights must be dimmed to that which is used during visual field testing. A light sensitive meter is used to calibrate the perimeter. This meter should be stored with the light sensitive side protected. The light meter is placed on the holder at the left side of the perimeter over the horizontal port. The meter will slide onto the holder. (This meter can be seen attached to the perimeter in Figure 6-3.) The flag in the holder is removed or pulled up out of the way so that the light can shine directly on the meter. (This step is very important so that 100% of the light will hit the meter.) To properly align the target light, insert field paper and locate the dot at 70 degrees on the chart paper (it is to the right of central fixation). The stylus on the pantograph arm is moved to this location and the arm locked into place by pushing the pin knob (located on the upper arm) into the locking hole. The arm will not move and the light will be projected directly onto the meter. To adjust the lighting, set the filter levers located on the back of the perimeter to the widest, brightest, and largest setting. (All levers will be moved to the right as in Figure 6-5.) The emitted light will be at its maximum projected level. The light shutter mechanism on the lower right side of the perimeter is rotated to provide a continual light beam. Check the reading on the meter. (A small light is provided near the light meter.) Adjust the knob (second knob in from the back of the machine on the lower left hand side) to achieve 1000 asb. Rotate the bulb, or replace it if neither side will achieve 1000 asb.

Once 1000 asb is achieved, replace or push the flag into position so that it is in the path of the directed light. The filter setting is moved from V4e to V1e. The flag's reflectance equals 31.5 asb. To view the target light, look through the horizontal port on the opposite side of the light meter. Some instruments have an eyepiece that must be adjusted to make the target clear. Adjust the bowl's reflectance by raising or lowering the movable shield over the bulbs housing (Figure 6-6). The illumination of the flag and the bowl must be the same. Raising the shield will darken the background, and lowering it will brighten the illumination. There are calibration marks on the shield that are used to compare readings. It is advisable to perform three readings to assure proper calibration. The three endpoints should not vary over 1 scale reading. Proper calibration will give a 31.5 asb light level. However, the scale may not read 31.5 asb because the light transmission of the bulb changes with use.

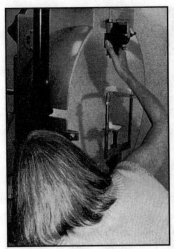

Figure 6-6. Raise or lower the movable shield over the bulbs housing to adjust bowl reflectance. (Reprinted from Blair B, Appleton B, Garber N, Crowe M, and Alven M. *Opticianry, Ocularistry and Ophthalmic Technology.* Thorofare, NJ: SLACK Incorporated; 1990.)

Automated Perimeter

Description and Purpose

An automated perimeter (Figure 6-7) is a fast, randomized visual field testing instrument utilizing several different stimuli that is similar to static perimetry. These automated versions monitor patient fixation, store patient data, and are programmed to identify probable defects. They are innovative in that most of the work is done for the perimetrist while keeping patient comfort at an optimum. Once the patient is prepared for the test, a few quick selections are made and the instrument records the patient's responses and prints out the test results. The subjective component is removed from the testing situation.

Maintenance

Keep the perimeter covered at night. The outside of the machine can be dusted with a soft cloth, but should not be directly sprayed with a cleaner. Maintenance for the Humphrey® Field Analyzer will be described here. Check manuals for other instruments. Do not use a dry cloth to clean the CRT. Electrostatic can build up causing instrument malfunction. Staticwipes are available from the manufacturer, but products can be purchased locally that are approved for use on this type of equipment (Endust™ for electronics). Wiping the CRT should be done at least once a month but more often in a dry climate. Remove jewelry and rings to prevent scratches on the bowl when cleaning. Care should be taken with long fingernails, and fingernail polish as well. The light pen tip can be cleaned using a cotton swab and alcohol. The patient response button should be cleaned with soap and water, alcohol, or a spray cleaner.

The automatic perimeter is a computer with disk drives. These drives should be cleaned at least three times a year depending on use. A disk drive cleaner is provided with the instrument and is simply inserted into the upper disk drive. The cleaning disk should be moistened with alcohol; a dry disk will damage the drive during cleaning. With the machine on, select DISK FUNCTIONS and press RECALL to start the cleaning cycle. At the end of the cleaning cycle, an error message will appear with the signal TRY AGAIN. Using the light pen press TRY AGAIN five times to end the cycle. Repeat the above procedure for the lower disk drive. To clean the tape

Figure 6-7. Humphrey®
Visual Field Analyzer.
(Photograph courtesy of
Zeiss Humphrey Systems
Inc.)

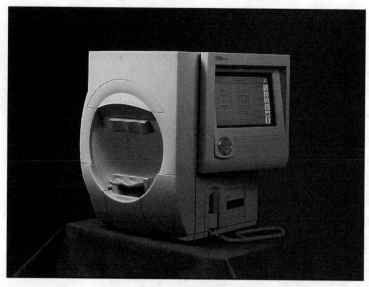

Figure 6-7. Humphrey®
Visual Field Analyzer.
(Photograph courtesy of
Zeiss Humphrey Systems
Inc.)

head, use a "mock" tape cartridge that has a cleaning pad, cleaning solution, and an arm for moving the cleaning pad across the head. Apply a few drops of the cleaning solution to the pad and insert it into the drive in the same fashion as a tape cartridge. Move the handle up and down to clean the entire head surface. Remove the cartridge and resume normal operation.

When a colored line appears at the edge of the field paper, it is at the end of the roll. To change the roll, turn the machine off. Push the open circles printed on the latches of the printer door and swing the door down. Remove the paper roll holder from the printer and remove the paper from the roll bar. Slip a new roll onto the roll bar so that the paper feeds from the top. Feed 6 inches of the paper through the printer (there is a diagram on the printer to use as a guide). Insert the paper holder into the printer, secure the fastener, feed extra paper through the printer door, and close it. Gently pull the paper to relieve any slack.

The printer ribbon must be changed when the print becomes light. Open the printer door and identify the ribbon cartridge. Pull on the top of the cartridge, lift the right end, and remove. Insert the new cartridge by inserting the left end and gently pushing in the right end; both ends will snap into place. Swing the printer back in and close the door.

The machine will give error messages when the projection or background illumination bulbs need replacing. To replace the projection bulb, turn the power off. The bulb is housed in the top back side of the machine. Open the access panel, and pull the bulb straight out. (Make sure that it is cool before handling.) Push in the new bulb using the protective envelope that the bulb comes in. Care should be taken not to touch the bulb because fingerprints will etch into the glass jacket. Close the access door. The two background illumination light bulbs are located near the front of the bowl at the two and nine o'clock positions. They are covered by a filter that can be rotated to expose the bulb. Push the bulb in and twist to remove.

Calibration

It is important to evaluate the stimulus of the perimeter once a week. The stimulus should have crisp edges. It should not look blurred or have inconsistencies in it. A visit from a service representative is necessary to change the condition of the stimulus.

Power Supply

The instrument uses a power cord that is plugged into a viable outlet. The fuse can be replaced if blown by first turning off the machine. Remove the power cord, slide the plastic cover to the left, and pull the fuse release tab. The fuse will pop out. Snap a new fuse into place and slide plastic cover back to the right. For a 120V instrument use a 4 amp, and for a 220V instrument use a 2 amp.

Instruments Used in the Retinal Exam

- Keep the ophthalmoscope set to the zero viewing lens to keep lenses clean.

- Turn instruments off to prolong battery and bulb life.

- A blast of canned air should be used regularly to keep all lenses dust-free.

- Never use regular tissues to clean delicate ophthalmic lenses.

- Never boil or autoclave ophthalmic lenses.

The instruments and equipment in this chapter are used to examine and treat the internal structures of the eye. These instruments are the direct ophthalmoscope, indirect ophthalmoscope, and contact and non-contact diagnostic and laser lenses.

Direct Ophthalmoscope

Description and Purpose

The direct ophthalmoscope (Figure 7-1) is a hand-held instrument used to view the internal structures of the eye. It contains a light source and a set of lenses that the observer can use to clearly focus the structures of the eye, particularly the retina. The view provided by the direct ophthalmoscope is monocular and non-stereoscopic. The view is upright (ie, not inverted) and its magnification is 14-15 times larger than normal.

Maintenance

The ophthalmoscope is a very delicate instrument. Care should be taken not to drop the instrument on a hard surface. Store the instrument with the viewing lenses set on zero. This moves all of the lenses to a position inside the instrument, keeping dust at a minimum. The lenses are set on disks, and are very small. It is difficult to clean these lenses, so this service should be performed by a professional. There are several types of ophthalmoscope bulbs and the type should be identified before changing. If the instrument contains a front surface mirror, clean it as described in Chapter 2.

Power Supply

See the power supply section for the retinoscope and follow similar procedures.

Indirect Ophthalmoscope

Description and Purpose

The indirect ophthalmoscope looks like a miner's cap that is worn on the head (Figure 7-2). Its optics provide a stereoscopic view of the retina. The light source is usually halogen. A diagnostic, condensing, aspheric lens is used in conjunction with the indirect ophthalmoscope. The stereoscopic view of the retina is inverted, reversed, and magnified 4-5 times larger than normal, with a 45 degree view. The periphery of the retina can be examined with the indirect ophthalmoscope. A scleral depressor (Figure 7-3) can be used to indent the sclera, allowing the examiner to see beyond the equator and out toward the ora serrata. The indirect ophthalmoscope is usually preferred over the direct for its larger field and stereoscopic view. It is the instrument of choice in retinal surgery.

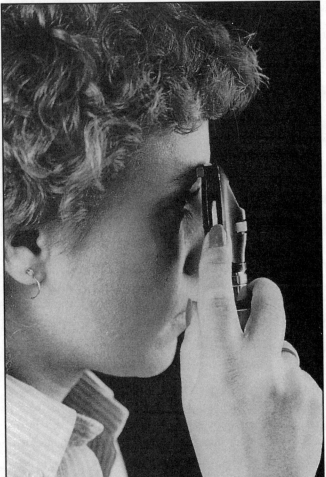

Figure 7-1. Direct ophthalmoscope. (Reprinted from Herrin MP. *Ophthalmic Examination and Basic Skills.* Thorofare, NJ: SLACK Incorporated; 1990.)

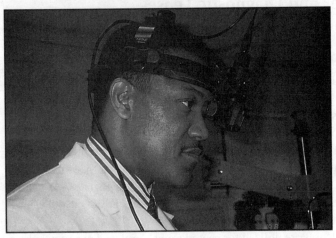

Figure 7-2. Indirect ophthalmoscope worn by a physician.

Figure 7-3. Scleral depressor.

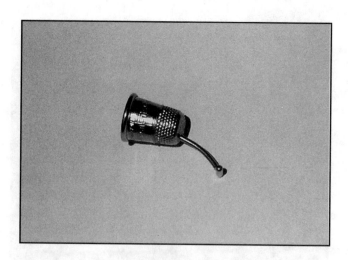

Maintenance

The indirect ophthalmoscope is hung on a provided hanger or placed in a case anchored to the wall. The eyepieces should be treated like any lens. A blast of canned air is used to remove dust and debris. If necessary, they can be wiped with alcohol for stubborn marks. The front surface mirror should be cleaned as described in Chapter 2. The bands can also be wiped with alcohol. There are cushions provided for comfort, and these can be removed from the bands and cleaned with soap and water. This should be performed more often if the instrument is used by more than one physician.

The bulb in the Heine Omega 180 and some other models is located in the bulb connector next to the cord connector. Pull the cord connector out and unscrew the bulb connector so that the bulb falls out. Replace with a new bulb, taking care not to touch the glass jacket. Check the bulb and bulb contacts and clean if necessary. Screw in bulb connector and replace the cord connector.

Laser and Diagnostic Lenses

Description and Purpose

Optical lenses (Figure 7-4) are very important and comprise a large portion of instruments used in eyecare. There are several types of lenses available on the market today. They can be used alone or incorporated into an instrument. There are lenses that must contact the eye, and those that do not. Lenses can be made of glass or plastic. The surface of the lens may be bloomed (coated with an anti-reflective coating). Many lenses have a yellow filter which provides patient comfort by removing blue, violet, and ultraviolet wavelengths, yet allowing the necessary longer wavelengths needed for fundus viewing. The diagnostic lenses (see also Figure 7-4) that are commonly used for fundus viewing with the indirect ophthalmoscope are the 20D to 40D lenses. With the slit lamp, the higher powered 60D to 90D lenses are used.

Laser and diagnostic contact lenses are utilized for central retinal, grid, and panretinal photocoagulation procedures. Special coatings (Argon and Diode laser/AR) provide optimal broadband transmission for outstanding resolution and unparalleled diagnostic and laser treatment capability. Some contact lenses are specially made to allow contact with the eye without the use of interface solutions.

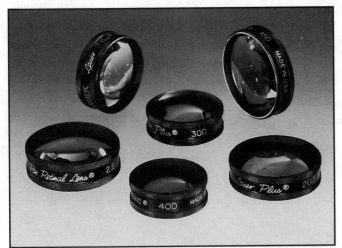

Figure 7-4. Optical lenses. (Photograph courtesy of Volk Optical Inc.)

Maintenance

Diagnostic lenses are precision optical instruments that deserve very meticulous care. The lens should be kept in its case when not in use. Lenses should not be touched because oils from the fingers will easily mark the surface. Always hold the lens by the mounting during use. A lens can become dislodged from its holder if too much cleaning solution is used, or due to general drying out over time. The lens can be re-attached by the manufacturer.

Clean lenses regularly to remove dirt, dust, and oily fingerprint smudges. To clean lenses that do not contact the eye, first remove dust and debris with canned air or a bulb syringe. Try a lens brush or lens paper to remove stubborn dust. Optical lens cleaners, solutions of four parts ether to one part alcohol, a half-and-half solution of ammonia and alcohol, as well as lint-free optical wipes are all available to clean non-contact lenses. Add the solution to a linen handkerchief that has been washed a number of times, or use a special optical lens wipe to clean the lens surface. Start in the center of the lens and, using a circular motion, work toward the outside of the lens. Do not rub the lens too hard, as this can remove the anti-reflective coating. Also, do not rub the lens with a dry cloth or wipe. This will promote dust buildup. To disinfect non-contact lenses, use alcohol or soak the lens for 20-25 minutes in a 2% aqueous solution of glutaraldehyde. To sterilize, use ethylene oxide gas (ETO) with aeration up to 150 degrees F. Standard ethylene oxide hospital sterilization procedures should be followed. Never autoclave or boil lenses.

To maintain lenses that touch the eye, rinse the lens after each use in tepid water to remove the interface solution and any tear film or mucus that may remain. A mild dishwashing liquid or contact lens cleaner can be used to clean the lens. Rinse the lens well to remove the soap or cleaner, and dry with a soft non-linting cloth. Never clean the contact surface element of these lenses with alcohol, hydrogen peroxide, or acetone because these chemicals can damage the lens surface. The anterior glass element can be cleaned regularly with lens cleaner.

To disinfect a diagnostic contact lens, soak in a 2% aqueous solution of glutaraldehyde for 20-25 minutes, or use a fresh solution of hypochlorite in a 1:10 dilution. Fill the lens cup holder and soak for 5-10 minutes. Either of these two methods must be followed by a thorough, brisk rinse with running water to remove the solutions. Dry with a lint-free cloth. To sterilize, use standard ethylene oxide gas procedures with aeration up to but not to exceed 130 degrees F. Never boil or autoclave these lenses.

Chapter 8

Instruments Used in the Contact Lens Exam

- Prolong bulb life by turning instruments off when not in use.

- Lock slit lamps when not in use.

- Check bulb contact points for corrosion on all instruments 2-3 times a year.

- Keratometers must have their calibration checked periodically.

- Fingerprints will dull the white rings of Placido's disk; care should be taken not to touch them.

The instruments and equipment in this chapter are used to determine the measurements needed in the fitting of contact lenses, including those used to measure the contact lens itself and its evaluation on the eye. These instruments are the slit lamp, Placido's disk, keratometer (ophthalmometer), corneal topography systems, radiuscope, lens modification unit, and lens diameter gauge.

OptT

OphA

CL

Slit Lamp

OptA

Description and Purpose

The slit lamp is one of the most important instruments used in the eyecare field. It is a biomicroscope that provides an illuminated, magnified, and stereoscopic view of the minute structures of the eye. There are two basic styles of slit lamps. The Haag-Streit and its copies have a vertical illumination source. The Zeiss and its copies have a horizontal prism reflected source (Figures 8-1a,b,c). Common to both types are a biomicroscope, a light source with various adjustments, various magnification settings, filters, a head rest, and a chin cup. Several attachments are available. These are a Hruby lens, an applanation tonometer, pachymeter, and photography equipment.

Maintenance

Keep the instrument covered at night to keep dust and debris at a minimum. Keep the instrument turned off when not in use. Canned air is useful to get dust out of the tiny crevices. The painted external parts of the instrument can be dusted with a soft lint-free cloth. Do not spray cleaning products on the instrument. This can damage moving parts, delicate lenses, and mirrors. The slit lamp has a locking device that should be engaged when the exam is completed. The instrument will roll when moving the slit lamp arm if not locked in place. If the slit lamp table is suddenly jerked and the slit lamp is not locked, it could be damaged.

The slit lamp has lenses and front surface mirrors that require the same care as described in Chapters 2 and 7. Lenses are cleaned with canned air, or a camel hair brush for stubborn debris. The front surface mirror on the Haag-Streit can be removed from its carrier. Grasp the sides of the mirror where it narrows near the top. Gently pull the mirror straight up. A lens wipe can be used to clean the mirror, or run a stream of water over the surface. Most of the water will roll off; the residual can be removed by patting the surface with a cotton swab or cloth. Do not rub the mirror or scratches will occur in the surface.

The chin rest and head rest can be wiped with a cleaner between patients. An alcohol wipe can be used, but care needs to taken to identify the type of material these parts are made out of. If the chin rest is rubber, the alcohol will ruin it. Also, excessive use of alcohol will dry out certain plastics. Some models have chin rest papers that can be changed between patients. Chin rest papers are replaced by removing the pin or screw that holds them in place, inserting new pack of papers, and replacing the anchor.

The slit lamp moves forward, backward, and side to side by the use of a joystick. The front to back movement is used for focusing. The instrument rolls on a ball bearing along a plastic gliding plate. Some slit lamps roll on running rails on each side of the instrument. The rails can be cleaned with a stiff brush. A buildup of dust and debris on the gliding plate will create drag and

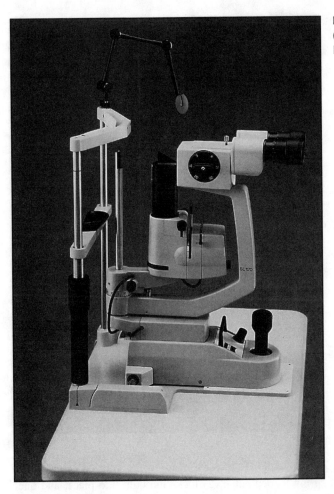

Figure 8-1a. Zeiss Slit Lamp SL 120. (Photograph courtesy of Zeiss Humphrey Systems Inc.)

slow the movement of the instrument. To clean the gliding plate, wipe the plate with an alcohol wipe. Move the instrument and note if there are any markings on the plate. The dirt from the ball bearing will leave a trail on the plate. Keep moving the slit lamp and wiping until no tracks remain. This can be done once or twice a year, depending on use. The alcohol can be drying to the plastic on the plate. Every five cleanings, spray a small amount of silicone or WD-40™ on the plate to keep it from cracking. This conditions the plastic and will also aid in slit lamp movement.

The main bulb on the slit lamp provides the illumination. Some instruments have a fixation device that also contains a bulb. Never touch the bulb, because fingerprints will etch into the glass jacket and prevent full illumination. Always unplug the instrument before attempting to change the bulb. The life of the bulb can be extended if the instrument is turned off after each use, and if the lowest voltage setting is selected when using the slit lamp.

The Haag-Streit's main bulb is housed at the top of the illumination tower. The housing case can be removed by loosening the two thumb screws on each side of the housing. The top is removed by pulling up so that the bulb and its base are exposed. The bulb can be lifted out of its housing and replaced with a new one. The bulb has a notch in it so that it will be properly placed in the housing. Be sure to check the contact points in the cover. Scrape contacts with an eraser or file if there is oxidation.

Figure 8-1b. Haag-Streit type slit lamp. (Photograph courtesy of Marco Technologies Inc.)

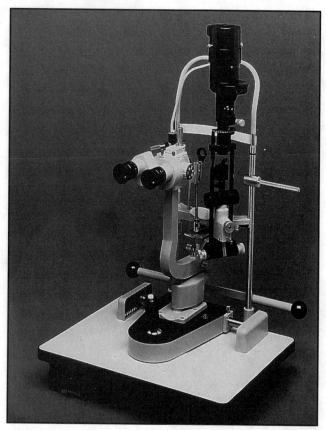

To replace the bulb on newer Zeiss models (Figure 8-2) loosen the knurled screw (1) to remove the lamp housing cover. A spring-loaded catch (2) locks the bulb into place, and once pressed, this catch unlocks the bulb so it can be removed. A new bulb (3) is placed in the lamp holder (4), and together they are pushing into the lamp opening. The catch will engage again and lock the bulb in place. The lamp housing cover is then put back into place and locked by tightening the knurled knob. The bulb of some of the older Zeiss models is in a housing that is removed by twisting the bulb holder and pulling down to expose the bulb. The bulbs are bayonet mounted. Once the bulb has been replaced, the holder is aligned by the white dots on the casing and pushed back into the housing. The holder is turned to the full extent to lock it and properly align the bulb correctly for full and even illumination.

Power Supply

The slit lamp is powered by electrical power cords. Check all connections to assure they are tight and attached to a viable source. Often the power cord is wired through the examination furniture. Occasionally check all connections and power cords.

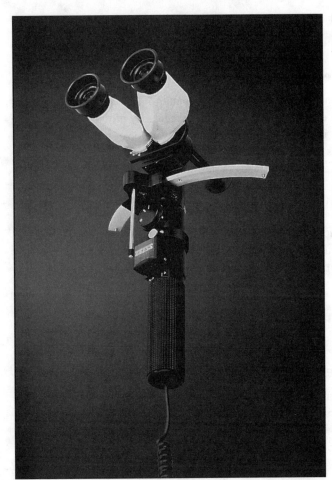

Figure 8-1c. Portable slit lamp HSO 10. (Photograph courtesy of Zeiss Humphrey Systems Inc.)

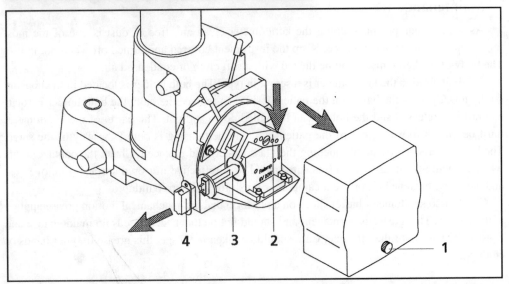

Figure 8-2. Replacing the bulb on the Zeiss slit lamp. (Illustration courtesy of Zeiss Humphrey Systems Inc.)

Placido's Disk

Description and Purpose

Placido's disk (Figure 8-3) is a round disk that has alternating black and white rings surrounding a small central hole. The disk is used to evaluate the regularity of the anterior surface of the cornea. Bright illumination is used behind the examiner who looks through the central aperture. The black and white rings are reflected off the patient's cornea and any distortions are noted. Placido's disk led to the development of the keratometer.

Maintenance

Keep the disk in a drawer. Do not touch the rings, as oils from the hands and fingers will dull the painted surface. Depending on the material of the disk, wipe with a soft cloth. If fingerprints appear, wipe gently with a slightly damp cloth to remove the marks.

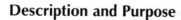

Keratometer (Ophthalmometer)

Description and Purpose

The keratometer, or ophthalmometer (Figure 8-4), is used to measure the curvature of the cornea's anterior central zone. These subjective measurements are commonly referred to as K-readings. These measurements are very important in contact lens fitting, determination of corneal astigmatism, and calculation of intraocular lens powers.

Maintenance

As with all equipment, keeping the keratometer clean and free of dust is one of the most important steps in its maintenance. Keep the instrument covered and turned off when not in use. The body of the keratometer can be dusted with a soft cloth or condensed air.

The bulb used in the keratometer is a screw-in type. The bulb holder is located in the housing on the lower part of the barrel on the patient's side. To replace the bulb, the bulb holder is rotated until it is released and the holder can be pulled down and out. The barrel of the keratometer must be moved forward (toward the patient) so that the housing is out of the way of the stage. The bulb is removed (without touching the glass jacket) and replaced. Check the contact points when changing the bulb. The bulb is surrounded by a reflective mirrored surface. Remove dust and debris with canned air or use a camel hair brush for stubborn buildup.

The Marco keratometer barrel slides on a platform that has mechanical motion grease applied at the factory. This grease is permanent and should not be touched. It needs no maintenance and is good for the life of the machine. Care should be taken not to get this grease on your hands or clothing.

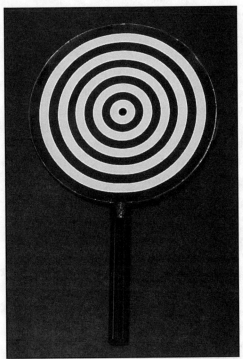

Figure 8-3. Placido's disk. (Photograph by Rhonda Curtis, COT, CRA.)

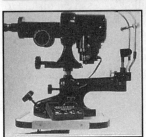

Figure 8-4. Keratometer with lensometer holder and calibrating ball in place. (Reprinted from Blair B, Appleton B, Garber N, Crowe M, and Alven M. *Opticianry, Ocularistry and Ophthalmic Technology.* Thorofare, NJ: SLACK Incorporated; 1990.)

Calibration

The calibration of the keratometer should be checked to assure accuracy of readings. Properly adjust the eyepiece before calibration and each use. Some manufacturers provide a test sphere(s). The test ball is set in place using a magnetic holder. Care should be taken not to get fingerprints on the spheres, because the oils can damage the surface and change the reading. A reading is taken with a chrome sphere of known radius. The machine is correctly calibrated if the reading taken matches the known radius. More than one measurement of different spheres should be taken if the readings are off more than .25D from the known radius. Do not attempt to adjust the drum scales, this must be done by the manufacturer. The barrel of the keratometer can become too tight or loose. Some machines have a screw that can be tightened or loosened to alleviate this problem. Great care should be taken when attempting this maneuver, because the washer for the screw can shift if not properly retightened.

Power Supply

Power is supplied by plugging the power cord into a viable outlet. Make sure that the connections are tight.

Automatic Keratometer

Description and Purpose

The automatic keratometer (Figure 8-5) is computerized like all other automatic equipment. The K-reading (measurement of the cornea's curvature) is obtained automatically by the machine. Some are hand-held like the Nidek KM-500 by Marco. This can be used with a battery pack or an A/C adapter. This unit takes the reading automatically when the mires are in focus. Readings appear on an LCD display, or can be transferred to an optional printer by infrared transmission. The instrument is hand-held or can be attached to a slit lamp.

Maintenance

Care should be taken when using the hand-held autokeratometer. The instrument should not be dropped or exposed to strong vibrations because damage can occur. The instrument should be kept in its case when not in use. The windows of the instrument should be kept away from bright illumination or sunlight. Measurements can be affected if fingerprints, dust, or dirt mark the measuring window. When the measuring and observation windows get dirty, they can be cleaned with compressed air, or an alcohol wipe can be used on stubborn dirt and debris. Clean the plastic parts of this instrument by wiping with a soft dry cloth. Do not spray cleaning solvents onto the instrument. A damp cloth may be used for stubborn dirt, taking care to not allow excessive moisture to seep into the instrument. If the instrument fails to work, do not attempt to open or disassemble it.

To replace the roll of paper in the printer, the roll is pulled out and the shaft is snapped out of its holder. The remaining paper is removed from the printer by pressing the paper feed button. A new roll is set in place with the outer side facing down. Feed the paper into the paper slot, press "Paper Feed," and it will automatically feed into the printer.

Power Supply

The autokeratometer has an attached battery pack that must be charged before use and then recharged overnight. The battery pack slides onto the bottom of the instrument by aligning the triangles on both the main body and the battery. The battery can be charged slowly with a trickle charge or quickly for a fast charge. A fast charge must be used when the low battery light comes on. (A fast charge connector is in the battery charger and is pulled out of the charger and attached to the battery when a fast charge is necessary.) Always recharge the battery with the proper charger. The battery can explode if charged with an improper charger or if it is thrown into a fire. The charging function will be damaged if the instrument is dropped in water. Do not pull on the cords of the A/C adapter; always remove cords by pulling on the plugs.

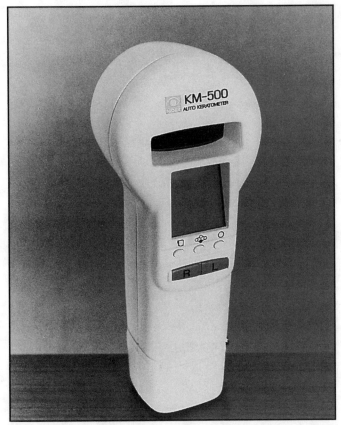

Figure 8-5. The KM-500 automatic keratometer. (Photograph courtesy of Marco Technologies Inc.)

Haag-Streit Ophthalmometer OM 900®

Description and Purpose

This ophthalmometer (Figure 8-6) automatically records the computerized K-reading on a display. The readings can also be printed. Javal markers (Figure 8-7) are moved into contact with each other for measurement.

Maintenance

Keep this instrument covered at night. Dust with a clean lint-free cloth. Clean stubborn dirt with a water-dampened cloth. Do not spray cleaners or water onto the machine. Keep the instrument away from any areas that might be exposed to a water aerosol. Glass surfaces can be brushed with a camel hair brush or wiped with a washed-out linen cloth if stubborn debris is present. If the instrument is not working properly no attempt should be made to open it.

Power Supply

The instrument has a power cord that must be securely attached to a viable socket. There are no fuses required.

Figure 8-6. Ophthalmometer OM 900® (Photograph courtesy of Haag-Streit.)

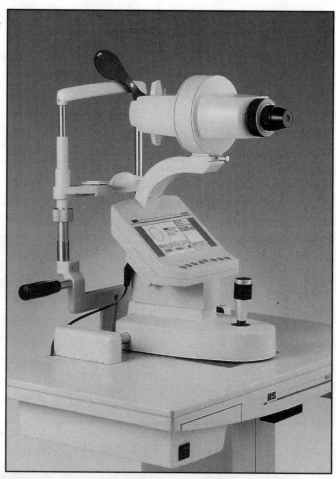

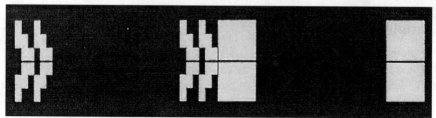

Figure 8-7. Javal markers. (Courtesy of Haag-Streit.)

Calibration

The instrument should have the calibration verified every year especially when it is used by several different people. A calibration device accompanies the instrument and is attached to the right-hand upright of the headrest. This device has several calibration nodules with specifically defined radii. The computer asks for known radii of the several nodules and calibration is performed on each. The instrument should be returned if it does not function properly after user calibration is performed.

Corneal Topography Systems

`CL`

Description and Purpose

The corneal topographer (Figure 8-8) is an electro-optical instrument that automatically analyzes and measures the shape of the cornea in fine detail. These measurements are very important when performing radial or photokeratotomy. The instrument consists of the optical cone and chin rest, a computer, monitor, printer, and power console.

Maintenance

The optical cone of this instrument has lighted rings that project onto the cornea, similar to a Placido's disk. The instrument should be covered at night to keep dust and debris off the instrument, especially the optical cone. The optical cone is a sensitive component and should not be touched or routinely cleaned. Lightly dust the instrument if needed, but take extra care while dusting around the optical cone. Never use alcohol or harsh detergents on the cone. The patient contact areas (chin and forehead rests) can be wiped with an alcohol wipe between patients. It is recommended that a servicing be scheduled once a year for a factory-trained representative to perform routine service and maintenance.

Power Supply

The power voltage is preset at the factory for 120V. The voltage must be changed before plugging in if your facility does not have a standard 120V grounded outlet.

Radiuscope

`CL`

Description and Purpose

The radiuscope, or gauge (Figure 8-9), is used to objectively determine the radius of a contact lens. Some can also determine lens thickness. It can measure convex or concave surfaces. Also, distortion or lens warpage can be detected with a radiuscope. The instrument consists of a body with an eyepiece that is very similar to a microscope. The radiuscope may have one or two eyepieces. It has a gauge that displays the measurement.

Maintenance

As with all equipment, keeping the radiuscope clean and free of dust is one of the most important steps in its maintenance. Keep the instrument covered when not in use. Turn it off when not in use to preserve the life of the bulb. The bulb is replaced by loosening the lamp socket set screws. The bulb is exposed when the housing is removed. Replace the bulb, then firmly and squarely replace lamp housing. This is very important because bulb alignment is critical for total field illumination. Most of the moving parts of the radiuscope are protected within the instrument's housing.

Optical surfaces should be treated as other precision lenses. Lens papers and solutions can be used to clean them.

Figure 8-8. The Alcon eyeSys Corneal Topography System.

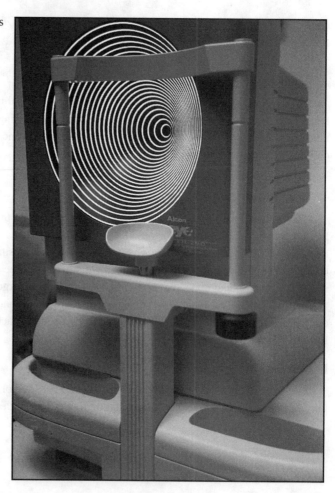

Power Supply

The radiuscope uses a power cord which is plugged into a standard grounded 120V A/C receptacle for its power supply.

Calibration

Always adjust the eyepiece(s) before using this instrument. To check the accuracy, use chrome spheres of known radius. If readings are off from the actual radii of the chrome balls, the instrument should be returned to manufacturer.

Lens Modification Systems

Description and Purpose

Gas permeable and traditional hard contact lenses can be modified using a lens modification system. A lens modification unit along with a well trained operator is essential in a busy contact

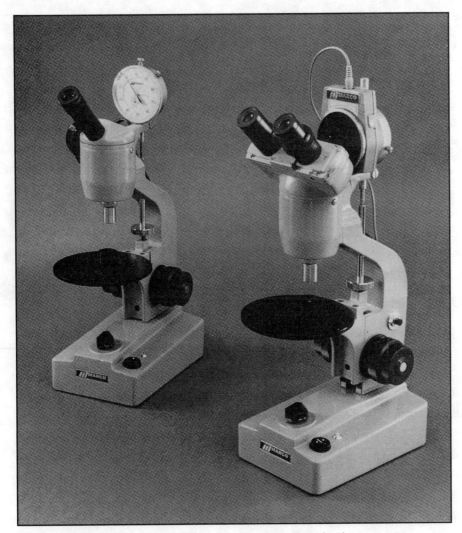

Figure 8-9. Radiusgauge. (Photograph courtesy of Marco Technologies, Inc.)

lens practice, as well as advantageous to the patient. This machine (Figure 8-10) is used to clean and polish contact lenses. It can also blend or add curves; flatten peripheral, intermediate or secondary curves; and change the contact lens' power. Contact lens edges can be reshaped, thinned, or blunted for better patient comfort. The machine uses multiple radius tools, and the spinner has various speeds (0 to 2000 rpm) for performing different modifications. Single speed models are also available.

Maintenance

The polisher is a simple machine. A splash tray covers and protects the motor and its components from contamination and corrosion from the polish. The tray can be easily removed and wiped clean depending on frequency of use. If the motor is broken, the entire unit can be replaced for a price almost comparable to replacing the motor.

Figure 8-10. Lens modification unit. (Photograph courtesy of Larsen Equipment Design.)

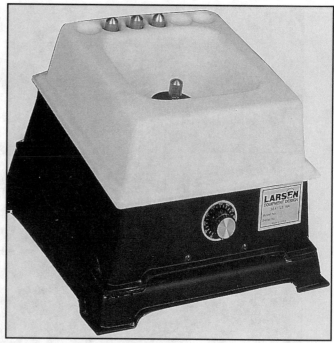

Power Supply

Attach the power cord to a viable wall outlet.

Lens Diameter Gauge (Loop)

Description and Purpose

This small, monocular magnifier with attached gauge (Figure 8-11) is used to measure the diameter of a contact lens. The lens is placed on the bottom plate of the gauge and the instrument is held up to the light. The diameter of the lens can be determined when placed against the grid.

Maintenance

Care should be taken not to drop the gauge on a hard surface. The gauge can be wiped with a soft, damp cloth, and dried.

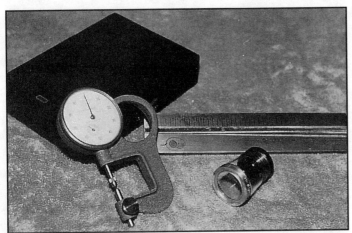

Figure 8-11. Lens thickness gauge, V-groove diameter gauge, and magnifying loupe. (Reprinted from Rakow PL. *Contact Lenses.* Thorofare, NJ: SLACK Incorporated; 1988.)

Chapter 9

Instruments Used in the Optical Lab

KEY POINTS

- Take care when warming plastic frames; do not overheat.
- Take care not to drop pliers, wrenches, or screwdrivers on a hard surface.
- Replace lens clock tip cover when not in use.
- Place instruments in cases or holders to protect from dust.

The following instruments are used in the optical shop to determine lens forms or size, make minor spectacle repairs, replace lenses, or make spectacle adjustments. These instruments are the frame warmer, optical pliers, screwdrivers, hex wrenches, lens clock, lens calipers and optical vernier, lens boxer, pupilometer, and edger.

Frame Warmer

Description and Purpose

Frame warmers are used to heat plastic frames for glazing, adjusting, or inserting lenses. There are two types—a salt pan (Figure 9-1a) and the hot air warmer (Figure 9-1b). The salt pan is a pan of glass beads or salt that is heated to a temperature range between 200 and 400 degrees F. Frames are placed into the pan and when properly heated, adjustments can be made in the plastic. The heat range of an air warmer is between 270 and 390 degrees F. The frame is held in the air warmer's heat stream until the plastic can be manipulated. The hot air warmer can save energy by eliminating the need to leave a frame warmer on all day.

Maintenance

The hot air frame warmer should not be placed near flammable materials or where water is used or stored. It should be turned on only when in use kept covered at night (when cool). It should not be used if the air flow opening is blocked, because it can damage the machine. Use canned air to remove accumulated dust, especially the inside dust cover.

Power Supply

The machine uses a grounded electrical cord that should be connected to 3-prong outlet. Unplug the machine if it is necessary to change the fuse. The fuse is removed by pushing in and turning the holder. Gently pull out, remove, and replace the fuse, 15 amp 250V. Push back in and rotate to lock the fuse in place.

Optical Pliers, Screwdrivers, and Hex Wrenches

Purpose and Description

Minor repairs of spectacles cannot be performed without a set of optical pliers, screwdrivers, and hex wrenches (Figure 9-2).

Maintenance

These are precision instruments that can last a lifetime if care is taken. Handle them gently and place in a holder when finished using.

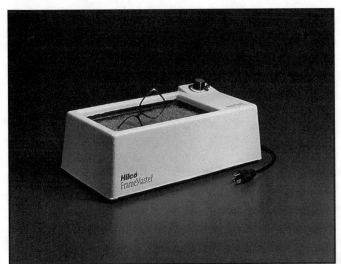

Figure 9-1a. Frame Master. (Photograph courtesy of Hilco®, a Division of Hilsinger.)

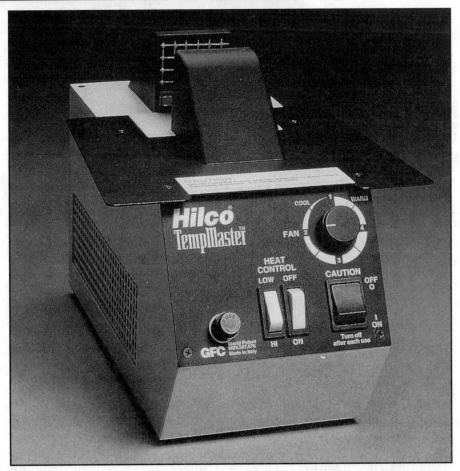

Figure 9-1b. Deluxe Hot Air Frame Warmer. (Photograph courtesy of Hilco®, a Division of Hilsinger.)

Figure 9-2. Hilco® pliers. (Photograph courtesy of Hilco®, a Division of Hilsinger.)

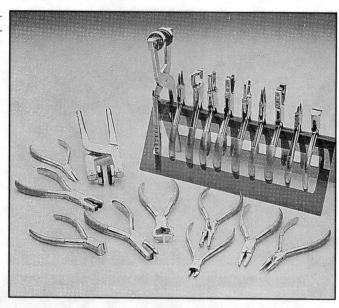

Lens Clock (Geneva Lens Measure)

Purpose and Description

The lens clock (Figure 9-3) is used to measure the base curve of a lens on either the front or back surface. The power of the lens can be calculated from this measurement. The lens clock can also determine which surface of the lens is the cylindrical surface, locate the axis of the cylinder, and establish the lens form. The same lens power can have many shapes or forms, therefore it is necessary to properly determine the lens form of the current prescription. The clock tips are placed on the lens surface and the base curve is read in quarter diopters from the instrument's dial.

Maintenance

The lens clock comes with a protective cap that protects the legs and tips from becoming damaged. Always replace the cap when the instrument is not in use. Care should be taken to not drop the clock on a hard surface.

Lens Thickness Calipers and Optical Vernier

Purpose and Description

Lens thickness calipers (see Figure 9-3) are used to determine the thickness of a spectacle lens. It looks like a pair of scissors and fits around the spectacle lens. Optical verniers (see Figure 9-3) are used for general measuring of inside and outside diameters of a lens.

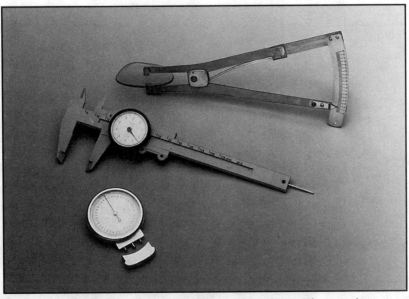

Figure 9-3. Gauge clock, calipers, and vernier by Hilco®. (Photograph courtesy of Hilco®, a Division of Hilsinger.)

Maintenance

Little maintenance is needed with the calipers and verniers. Replace in a case or drawer when finished using and take care not to drop these instruments on a hard surface.

Lens Boxer

Description and Purpose

The lens boxer (Figure 9-4) is a simple gauge that is used in the optical shop to quickly determine a lens' physical measurements. When placed in the boxer, the height and width can be measured. The bifocal height and inset can also be determined.

Maintenance

Keep the boxer in a drawer to keep it dust-free when not in use.

Pupilometer or Pupil Gauge

Description and Purpose

The pupilometer, or pupil gauge (Figure 9-5), is an instrument used to measure interpupillary distance (IPD). A light source provides a corneal reflex that is used to accurately determine the IPD.

Figure 9-4. Hilco® boxer. (Photograph courtesy of Hilco®, a Division of Hilsinger.)

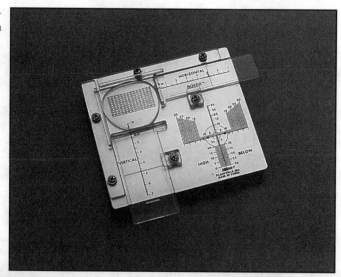

Figure 9-5. Measuring IPD using the pupilometer.

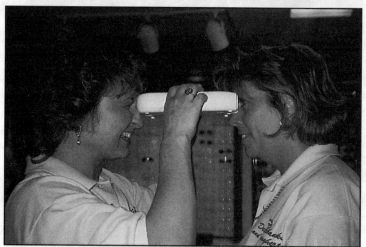

The examiner can line up the reflexes and be assured of an accurate reading. The pupilometer is very helpful and much more accurate in cases of an extremely large IPD and anisocoria.

Maintenance

The pupilometer is a sensitive instrument and should not be dropped. The outside body can be wiped with a damp cloth. The forehead and nose rest should be wiped with an alcohol wipe between patients.

There is a bulb inside that may need to be replaced. Some units have a built-in bulb and must be returned to the manufacturer to replace a blown bulb.

Power Source

Most pupilometers run on standard AA or AAA batteries.

Edger

Description and Purpose

The edger (Figure 9-6) is used to grind uncut lens blanks to fit the size and shape of a frame. Edgers have basically remained the same over the years, but vast improvements have been made in wheel types and construction. Most edgers today have a diamond wheel. Older models have two motors, while newer models can have up to four. Each motor controls a different movement. Some edgers require patterns to grind lenses while others are patternless. The characteristics are very different from machine to machine. Check the manual for proper maintenance. The following is a guide for the Grande Mark Bevel Edger.

Maintenance

Keeping an edger maintenance schedule is very important. The machine should be regularly checked, adjusted, and cleaned to maintain quality performance. A more thorough maintenance, including calibration check and coolant changes, can be performed on a regular weekly basis. This would also depend on the number of jobs performed each day. Debris from lens grinding should be kept at a minimum. The edger will last longer if kept very clean. During grinding, debris is carried off by water that passes through screens and filters. These need meticulous attention and frequent cleaning. The outside surface can be washed with a mild soapy detergent. The inside wheel and housing assembly can be wiped with a damp cloth, or debris can be blown away with a low pressure hose or canned air. Water can also be used to remove stubborn debris. Proper care should be taken to protect eyes from flying debris during cleaning and regular use. Some parts, especially splash guards, can be removed for cleaning if accumulation is heavy.

Lubrication is crucial to the moving parts. A lightweight oil should be used once a week (or every other week, depending on usage) to allow trouble-free operation. Lubricate all hinges, gears, and ball bearings. Although lubrication is important, too much oil or grease can help to accumulate dirt and debris.

Most wheels are bonded or electroplated diamond wheels. Do not attempt to stone or clean an electroplated diamond wheel. This can only be cleaned with a stiff bristle brush and an abrasive (such as Ajax™ or Comet™). The bonded diamond wheel needs to be stoned when it looks coated or when it takes longer than usual to edge a lens. Two stones are usually available to sharpen the wheel. These stones need to be soaked in coolant before use. To stone the roughing wheel, unplug the power to the coolant and turn the machine on to get the wheel to full speed. (Some machines require that the coolant and water remain running.) Then turn the power off and place the white stone against the wheel to clean it. The stone will stop. Repeat this process two or three more times. The gray stone is used to stone the finishing or bevel wheel. This is not needed very often. Leave the coolant running and bring the wheels to full speed. Depress the gray stone to the wheel for a few seconds. Turn the wheel off; repeat if necessary.

Coolant is added to the water to reduce the heat generated by the edging process, to remove debris, and to reduce lens chipping and cracking. The coolant also provides a certain lubricating effect and is important in maintaining wheel life. The coolant should be changed once a week depending on use. The coolant may need to be changed more often when grinding plastic lenses. Coolants come in different strengths, so the proper mixture must be used. The coolant is usually located in a large tank below the edger. To replace the coolant, drain it from the machine, then

Figure 9-6. Edger. (Photograph courtesy of AIT Industries.)

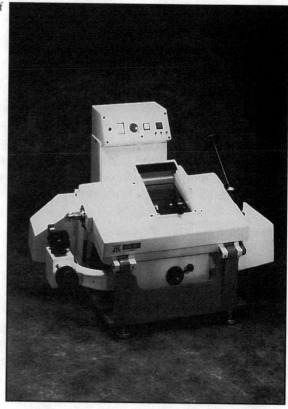

clean the coolant pump and all areas before replacing. Keeping sludge and debris to a minimum prolongs machine life.

The bevel placement can be changed using a special tool from the manufacturer. The bevel should first be examined to determine if it is too far right or left. Turn the coolant off. Bring the wheel to full speed and place the bevel placement tool to the side of the V that is removing too much bevel.

Retruing a diamond bonded wheel must be performed often when grinding a fair amount of glass lenses. This retruing is needed when the wheel does not produce a sharp bevel. Some machines have a retruing tool for minor adjustments. If the finishing wheel is worn too round or the V is worn too deep, the wheel should be returned to the manufacturer for retruing.

Proper care is needed for the right-hand spindle felt pad. This pad insures proper lens size and shape. After 1200 or so lenses, the pad will be thin and worn and must be replaced. The pad is on the adapter. Using some form of heat (match, lighter, or salt pan) warm the adapter and remove the old pad. Use cement glue to attach the new pad. The pad must be allowed to dry for 20-30 minutes, or the pad can be held in place by a blocked lens overnight.

Some machines use finger guides which must be replaced when the right edge (which is normally straight) has developed a curve. This guide is replaced to maintain positive control of bevel placement.

Power Supply

Insert the power cord plug into a viable AC outlet. Ensure that all connections are tight. The Grande Mark Bevel Edger has five fuses, four on the rear control panel and one near the power plug.

Chapter 10

Maintenance of Specialized Instruments

- Cover instruments or keep in cases when not in use.

- Do not attempt to repair photography equipment.

- Do not store pachymeter on slit lamp. Put in its case when not in use.

- Do not drop these delicate instruments!

The instruments and equipment in this chapter are occasionally used, not routinely, in eyecare. These instruments are the exophthalmometer, pachymeter, ophthalmodynamometer, ultrasound, and photography equipment.

Exophthalmometer

Description and Purpose

The exophthalmometer (Figure 10-1) is an instrument that is used to measure enophthalmos and exophthalmos, two conditions commonly seen in thyroid eye disease or orbital trauma. The exophthalmometer consists of a bar with movable carriers containing mirrors and a measuring scale on each side. Older models are made of metal, while newer models are plastic and very lightweight.

Maintenance

Little maintenance is required for the exophthalmometer. The instrument comes in a carrying case and should remain in its case when not in use. Care should be taken not to drop or bend the instrument. The exophthalmometer can be washed and dried with a soft damp cloth. Alcohol wipes should be used on the edges that are exposed to the patient's skin. The mirrors in the carriers are front surface mirrors and should be cared for as described in Chapter 2. Too much cleaning solution can cause the mirrors to become loose. Super Glue™ can be used to reattach the mirrors.

No power source or calibration is needed.

Ophthalmodynamometer

Description and Purpose

The ophthalmodynamometer is an instrument used to give an approximate measurement of the relative pressures in the central retinal arteries, and is an indirect means of assessing carotid artery flow. The instrument is pen-shaped and can either have a dial or a plunger scale to indicate readings. It is commonly used in the diagnostic workup of carotid insufficiency, thrombosis, and stenosis. It has sometimes been used as a research tool in glaucoma comparing episcleral venous pressure to intraocular pressure.

Maintenance

The ophthalmodynamometer is a delicate instrument that should not be dropped. It comes in a carrying case and should remain in it when not in use. The foot that is placed on the eye during the exam is metal, and should be wiped with an alcohol swab then thoroughly dried between patients.

There is no power source or need for calibration.

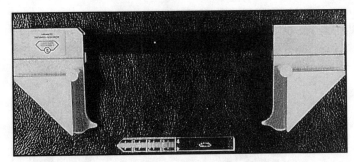

Figure 10-1. Exophthalmometer. (Reprinted from Blair B, Appleton B, Garber N, Crowe M, Alven M. *Opticianry, Ocularistry and Ophthalmic Technology.* Thorofare, NJ: SLACK Incorporated; 1990.)

Pachymeter

Description and Purpose

The pachymeter (Figure10-2) is an instrument used to measure corneal thickness. The pachymeter that is attached to the slit lamp consists of two plano glass plates on top of each other edge-to-edge. The beam from the slit lamp is divided through the pachymeter and the top plate can be rotated for measurement. The epithelium and endothelium are used as measuring points. Digital units are self-contained (ideal for operating rooms) and have a probe that automatically reads the thickness.

Mentor's Advent™ pachymeter is an advanced digital pachymeter which provides both lamellar and corneal bed measurements, making it particularly valuable to the LASIK surgeon. It will of course make conventional corneal thickness measurements. It also provides for up to eight templates or patterns of measurements, allowing a thorough mapping of the corneal thickness.

Maintenance

The slit lamp attached model is a delicate instrument that should be kept in its case. To remove dust and debris, attach it to the slit lamp and use canned air.

The digital pachymeter should be covered at night and turned off when not in use. Keep the probe secure in its holder; do not let it come into contact with extreme heat or allow it to strike a hard surface. Keep the cable coiled in its holder, and do not allow it to get pinched when opening and closing the console. The outside case can be wiped with a soft cloth to prevent dust build-up. Care should be taken when wiping the LCD screen because heavy pressing and scratching can damage it.

The probe tip should be cleaned with an alcohol wipe between patients. If sterilization is needed the probe can be gas sterilized with ethylene oxide (EtO). Cold sterilizing equivalents can also be used on the tip. Autoclaving the probe will damage it.

A red warning strip appears on the paper when a new roll is needed. The paper chamber door will spring up when the latch is slid toward the front. Push the paper release lever down to release the old roll. Insert the paper roll axil into the new roll and place it into the paper well. The paper should roll out from underneath. Pull the paper out and up over the well and feed it through the exit slot. Flip the lever back up and replace the paper well cover.

Power Supply

A power cord must be attached to a viable wall socket. Two fuses are located on the rear panel. Use 2 amp 5x20 with the 120V instrument and 1 amp 5x20 with the 220V instrument. To

Figure 10-2. Advent™ Pachymeter. (Photograph courtesy of Mentor® O&O.)

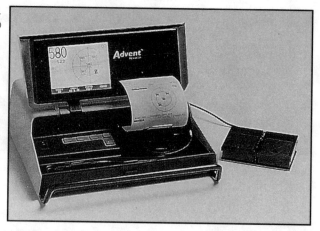

change fuses, unplug the instrument. Gently remove the fuse holder using a screwdriver until it snaps out. Remove the old fuse, insert the new one, and reinsert the fuse holder.

Ultrasonic Instruments

Description and Purpose

Ultrasound units utilize high frequency waves to create diagnostic imaging to measure the axial length of the eye, detect ocular pathology, measure structure thickness, and locate foreign bodies in the eye. The two most commonly used in the ophthalmic field are the A and B scans. The A-scan (biometry) is a single dimensional display that shows the amplitude and spacing of echoes. It measures the axial length of the eye for IOL power calculation. The B-scan (diagnostic imaging) is a two dimensional display that shows the different brightness of various echoes. It shows a cross-sectional view of the eye and its structures. There are instruments (Figure 10-3) that can obtain both A and B scan measurements, or there are separate instruments available to perform either test.

Maintenance

The following maintenance information describes the Mentor Advent™ A/B system. Users of other instruments should consult maintenance manuals. Cover the instrument at night to keep surfaces free of dust and debris. It should be placed in a cool, dry place to protect the electronic parts. Non-linting cloths can be used to clean the high resolution CRT monitor screen. Lightly dust the keyboard with compressed air. Do not spray solvents directly onto the instrument.

There are two separate probes used with the dual function instrument. The A-scan probe touches the cornea and must be cleaned in with isopropyl alcohol between patients. The alcohol must evaporate thoroughly before applying the probe to the patient's eye. The probe is hand-held, but can also be attached to the slit lamp. The B-scan probe most often touches the closed eyelid. It too should be cleaned with alcohol after rinsing the probe with saline to remove ultrasound transmission gel. Do not autoclave probes. Do not immerse the probe's cable or metal connector. Allow to dry if the probe becomes wet before use. If the instrument fails to work properly, return to manufacturer for repairs.

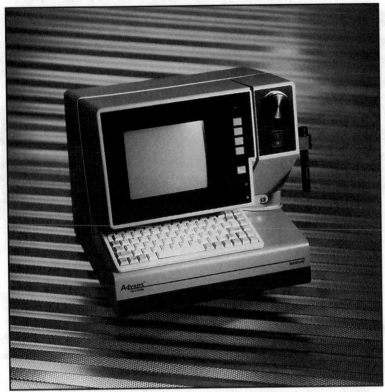

Figure 10-3. Advent™ A/B scan. (Photograph courtesy of Mentor® O&O.)

Power Supply

Plug the power supply cord into the instrument and to a viable wall socket. Two fuses help to protect the electronic circuitry. To replace, remove the power cord from the rear instrument panel. Pull out the fuse carrier by pushing down on the small tab in the middle of the carrier and pulling the carrier out. Remove old fuses and replace with new 5 mm x 20 mm Type T 2.AL, 250V fuses.

Fundus Camera

`OptT`
`OphT`
`RA`

Description and Purpose

The fundus camera (Figure 10-4) first became commercially available in 1926 for documentation of the retina; however, it was not until the electronic flash was adapted for use in the fundus camera and a paper was published describing the technique used for intravascular injection of fluorescein and retinal photography, that fundus photography and retinal angiography became a standard diagnostic procedure for ophthalmologists. These events occurred in the late 1950s and early 1960s.

The fundus camera is a low powered microscope utilizing an aerial image system of focusing and equipped with a 35mm camera back. It is positioned on a height adjustable table with chin and forehead rests for patient support and positioning. It has a joystick control for camera positioning and a camera height adjustment. Fundus cameras equipped for fluorescein angiography have a barrier and exciter filter positioned in the optical light path, and a power supply adequate

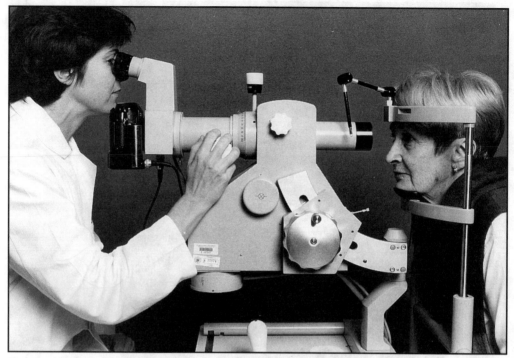

Figure 10-4. Fundus camera. (Reprinted from Cunningham D. *Clinical Ocular Photography*. Thorofare, NJ: SLACK Incorporated; 1998.)

for rapid sequence photography. Most fundus units also come equipped with green filters in the 540-570 nm range for so-called red-free photography. The newer digital units are also equipped with infrared filter sets for Indocyanine Green Angiography, used in computerized imaging.

Maintenance

Daily maintenance of the fundus camera is important. Cover the instrument at night. The instrument should be kept clean and can be wiped with a soft cloth. Do not spray cleaning solutions on the exterior of the machine. The plastic parts such as the forehead and chin rests should be disinfected after each patient by cleaning as recommended by OSHA guidelines.

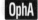

Cleaning the Lens

The lens of the camera should be kept covered whenever photography is not being performed. Removal of dust particles on the front lens element can be done by using a rubber-ball blower (such as a ear syringe). Care should be taken in using canned air because it may put a coating of freon on the lens. If fingerprints or smudges necessitate further cleaning of the front lens, use a moist lint-free lens tissue (or cotton) and denatured alcohol, or a mixture of denatured alcohol and acetone. The cleaner should never be put directly on the lens, but only a small quantity on the tissue or cotton. Do not touch the lens with the section of tissue or cotton that has been in contact with your hands, as deposits may be transferred to the lens. Starting at the center of the lens, gently wipe the lens surface in ever-widening circles to the edge of the lens. Discard the tissue and repeat with clean tissue and cleaner. Repeat this process as necessary. It is important to never rub the lens, as some lenses are coated and the anti-reflective coating can be removed by too vigorous a cleaning. After cleaning in this manner, it may be necessary to remove dust or lint particles from the lens by blowing with the blower ball or using an antistatic lens brush. If using an anti-static lens brush, be sure to never touch the bristles. Deposits from your hands may transfer to the bristles and then spread onto the lens surface. The rear lens element and internal optics should only be cleaned by an authorized service representative from the manufacturer.

Viewing Lamp

Check the owner's manual to locate the viewing lamp of your unit. The Zeiss' lamp is located on the right side of the unit; the Topcon's lamp is located inside and to the left.

Check to make sure the power is off and power cord is unplugged. Follow the instructions in the owner's manual and remove the old lamp. (Be sure that the lamp has cooled before touching.) When replacing the new lamp be sure there are no spots or fingerprints on it, as these may decrease its life. Wrap the lamp in tissue or foam to insert. After inserting the new lamp, assemble the unit and put viewing on the lowest level of intensity before turning the power on. Gradually increase the intensity until the maximum level is reached. This allows for a gradual warm-up of new bulbs.

Flash Tube

Xenon flash tubes in fundus units need to be replaced not only when they stop flashing, but also when inconsistent flashes occur or when images appear underexposed at the normal settings. A darkened area or whitish deposits on the glass tube can be seen when tubes are in need of replacement. Follow instructions outlined in the owner's manual to locate and replace the tubes. Since these tubes can hold a charge, it is important to be sure the power to the unit is off and the power cord unplugged. Wait for at least 5 minutes after the unit is off before changing tubes. Never put any metal objects or material that could conduct a charge near the flash tube. It is extremely important that the tube be replaced properly in order to assure the alignment of the optics. It is highly recommended that an extra flash tube be kept on hand for each camera. Log the date the new tube was inserted for future reference. This can be helpful to estimate the life of the tube or to determine whether or not the tube itself was faulty. The flash intensity and number of flashes will affect the life of the tube. It is advisable to visually check the tubes for deposits annually.

Power Supply

Insert the power cord into a viable outlet. Ensure that all connections are tight. Each fundus camera has a power unit with fuses. Check the owner's manual to find out where these fuses are located. Make sure that spare fuses are available. When checking a fuse, press down on the fuse holder and remove it by rotating counter-clockwise. If the fuse is bad, the filament will be darkened or broken. If there is any doubt, replace it with a new fuse. The fuses control different operations of the fundus unit and it is advisable to check the fuses first before changing tubes or viewing lamps.

Bibliography

Blair B, Appleton B, Garber N, Crowe M, Alven M, *Opticianry, Ocularistry and Ophthalmic Technology*. Thorofare, NJ: SLACK Incorporated; 1990.

Cleaning, Disinfection & Sterilization. Mentor, Ohio: Volk Optical, Inc; 1996.

The Goldmann Contact Glasses. Koeniz, Switzerland: Haag-Streit AG.

Herrin, MP. *Ophthalmic Examination and Basic Skills*. Thorofare, NJ: SLACK Incorporated; 1990.

Hilco® Lens Clock Owner's Manual. Plainville, Mass: Hilco®, a Division of Hilsinger; 1992.

Hilco® TempMaster™ Deluxe Hot Air Frame Warmer Instructions. Plainville, Mass: Hilco® a Division of Hilsinger; 1993.

Instruction and Interpretation Manual, MTI Photoscreener™. Lancaster, Pa: Medical Technology & Innovations, Inc; 1996.

Instruction Handbook, Lensmeter. Jacksonville, Fla: Marco Technologies, Inc.

Instruction Handbook, Keratometer. Jacksonville, Fla: Marco Technologies, Inc.

Instruction Manual, Advent™ A/B Scan. Santa Barbara, Calif: Mentor® O&O Inc.

Instruction Manual, Advent™ Pachymeter. Santa Barbara, Calif: Mentor® O&O Inc.

Instruction Manual, Brightness Acuity Tester. Jacksonville, Fla: Marco Technologies, Inc.

Instruction Manual, Goldmann Perimeter. Koeniz, Switzerland: Haag-Streit Inc.

Instruction Manual, Humphrey® Visual Field Analyzer. Dublin, Calif: Zeiss Humphrey Systems Inc.

Instruction Manual, KM-500 Hand-Held Auto Keratometer. Jacksonville, Fla: Marco Technologies, Inc.

Instruction Manual, Keratometer. Jacksonville, Fla: Marco Technologies, Inc.

Instruction Manual, Lenschek™ Advanced Logic Lensmeter®. Buffalo, NY: Reichert Ophthalmic Instruments, a Division of Leica; 1994.

Instruction Manual, Lensmeter. Jacksonville, Fla: Marco Technologies, Inc.

Instruction Manual, Nidek RT 2100 Auto Refractor. Jacksonville, Fla: Marco Technologies, Inc.

Instruction Manual, Ophthalmometer OM 900® Koeniz, Switzerland: Haag-Streit Inc; 1997.

Instruction Manual, Model 30 Classic™ Pneumatonometer. Santa Barbara, Calif: Mentor® O&O Inc.

Instruction Manual, Perkins Hand-Held Applanator. Koeniz, Switzerland: Haag-Streit Inc.

Instruction Manual, SL 120. Dublin, Calif: Zeiss Humphrey Systems Inc.

Instruction Manual, Titmus 2a Vision Screener. Petersburg, Va: Titmus Optical, Inc.

Instruction Manual, Tono-Pen™ XL. Santa Barbara, Calif: Mentor® O&O Inc.

Instruction Manual, Ultramatic RXMaster™ Phoropter®. Buffalo, NY: Reichert Ophthalmic Instruments, a Division of Leica; 1994.

Instruction Manual, Visual Acuity Projector. Jacksonville, Fla: Marco Technologies, Inc.

Instruction Manual, XPERT™ NCT™ PLUS, Advanced Logic Tonometer. Buffalo, NY: Reichert Ophthalmic Instruments, a Division of Leica; 1994.

Kendall, CJ. *Ophthalmic Echography*. Thorofare, NJ: SLACK Incorporated; 1990.

Ledford, JK, Sanders, VN. *The Slit Lamp Primer*. Thorofare, NJ: SLACK Incorporated; 1998.

Stein HA, Slatt BJ, Stein RM. *The Ophthalmic Assistant, 6th ed*. St. Louis, Mo: Mosby; 1994.

User's Guide, Humphrey® Visual Field Analyzer. Dublin, Calif: Zeiss Humphrey Systems Inc; 1997.

Index

For your information

This book and many others on numerous different topics are available from SLACK Incorporated. For further information or a copy of our latest catalog, contact us at:

Professional Book Division
SLACK Incorporated
6900 Grove Road
Thorofare, NJ 08086 USA
Telephone: 1-609-848-1000
1-800-257-8290
Fax: 1-609-853-5991
E-mail: orders@slackinc.com
WWW: http://www.slackinc.com

We accept most major credit cards and checks or money orders in US dollars drawn on a US bank. Most orders are shipped within 72 hours.

Contact us for information on recent releases, forthcoming titles, and bestsellers. If you have a comment about this title or see a need for a new book, direct your correspondence to the Editorial Director at the above address.

*If you are an instructor, we can be reached at the address listed above or on the Internet at **educomps@slackinc.com** for specific needs.*

Thank you for your interest and we hope you found this work beneficial.